The International Behavioural

T0227902

ADMISSION TO RESIDENTIAL CARE

TAVISTOCK

The International Behavioural and Social Sciences Library

HEALTH & SOCIETY
In 12 Volumes

ADMISSION TO RESIDENTIAL CARE

PAUL BREARLEY
WITH FRANK HALL, PENNY
GUTRIDGE, GLENYS JONES AND
GWYNETH ROBERTS

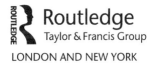

Routledge
Taylor & Francis Group

LONDON AND NEW YORK

First published in 1980 by
Tavistock Publications Limited

Published in 2001 by
Routledge
2 Partk Square, Milton Park, Abingdon, Oxfordshire OX14 4RN
711 Third Avenue, New York, NY 10017

First issued in paperback 2014

Routledge is an imprint of the Taylor and Francis Group, an informa business

British Library Cataloguing in Publication Data
A CIP catalogue record for this book
is available from the British Library

Admission to Residential Care
ISBN 0-415-26428-6
Health & Society: 12 Volumes
ISBN 0-415-26509-6
The International Behavioural and Social Sciences Library
112 Volumes
ISBN 0-415-25670-4

ISBN 13: 978-1-138-86741-3 (pbk)
ISBN 13: 978-0-415-26428-0 (hbk)

Admission to Residential Care

Paul Brearley,

WITH
Penny Gutridge, Frank Hall,
Glenys Jones, Gwyneth Roberts

TAVISTOCK PUBLICATIONS
LONDON and NEW YORK

First published in 1980 by
Tavistock Publications Ltd
2 Park Square, Milton Park, Abingdon, Oxon, OX14 4RN

Published in the USA by
Tavistock Publications
in association with Routledge.
270 Madison Ave, New York NY 10016

Typeset by Scarborough Typesetting Services

British Library Cataloguing in Publication Data
Brearley, Paul
Admission to residential care. — (Residential
social work).
1. Institutional care — Great Britain
2. Inmates of institutions — Great Britain
I. Title   II. Series
361'.05   HV245   80-40556

ISBN 0-422-76930-4
ISBN 0-422-76940-1 Pbk

Contents

General Editor's Foreword

Admitting people to some form of residential care for long, medium, or short periods of time, has been with us for a very long time. The range of such caring situations is wide, and across this spectrum various special approaches have developed ranging from containment to treatment and including many based upon specific theories of human behaviour and the socializing processes.

Such diversity contains large elements of tradition and little experimentation. Because of the fact that many residential situations are regarded as 'last resort' approaches, the people who work in them are not often regarded as professionals nor considered to need much in the way of training. There are exceptions to these statements where, in specific areas of human difficulty, usually relating to some form of mental disturbance, great efforts have been made to use skilled staff and designed environments to produce maximum beneficial effect. The expertise developed as a result of these efforts has not often spread to the wider sphere of which they are a part, probably for two main reasons: a) such successful experiments are often very costly in time, skilled personnel, and money; and b) there is little realization of the need for such a level of performance nor acceptance of the responsibility to provide it.

This situation is clearly marked in the production of material which could be considered to be valuable to those engaged in the practice of residential care. There is literature which discusses the wider theoretical issues of placing people in residential institutions, there is a small number of books concerned with residential practice in very specific areas of concern, for example prisons and hospitals, and an even smaller number concerned with the principles of such practice. Courses for people engaged in this care practice are few and in general the picture is one of gross understimulation and fairly massive lack of support and understanding.

Such information as is available then, tends to be specific, related to a special situation, and not easily extrapolated to provide guidelines for others to follow. But it must be reasonably obvious to anyone looking at residential care dispassionately, that all the apparently dissimilar practices gathered under this wide banner have many very fundamental characteristics in common. The most obvious of these is that all start from the situation of change – the removal of individuals either voluntarily or compulsorily from one form of accommodation to another, the latter thought generally to be designed to meet given deficiences in the person's former life style.

This series has been created to bring before all those interested in residential care the experience of practitioners, consultants, teachers, and researchers which will highlight methods, approaches, and models of practice, of which they have first-hand experience, and relate these to residential care in general.

Admission to Residential Care deals with one of the most basic of the characteristics that exists in the residential situation, the transition from one state of accommodation to another. The factors involved in making the transition are clearly outlined here, starting from the decision that such a move may be necessary in the interests of the client. The authors consider all the data which should be included in the decision and introduce the concept of 'risk' which is a recurring theme throughout the book.

Having considered the general problems of risk-taking decisions, the authors look at this process in relation to the admission to care of children, the mentally ill, and the elderly. The consequences of bad decisions for the client, the others involved, and the providers of resources are considered in some detail.

Although ideal performance is considered here as a guide, it is also clearly recognized by all the authors that reality often imposes severe limitations upon the resources available and adds an extra element of risk in that choice has to be made between possibilities which meet the need at a level often well below that which is desirable and necessary.

The part which legislation plays in admission procedures is often crucial, defining the reasons for proceeding but seldom specifying means or methods and frequently making little allowance for situations which are individual and personal.

The authors have tried to bring some order into the chaotic and frequently emotional issues surrounding the admission to care — a difficult task. In so far as they have succeeded it is due to their personal experience and an ability to relate it to a wider set of issues than the immediate concern. There is some evidence that the quality of an admission procedure, as seen by those involved, has a lasting effect on the subsequent process of care and its outcome. This being so this detailed consideration of admission is not only timely but essential for all those interested in residential care.

TOM DOUGLAS
March 1980

Preface

This book includes chapters from a number of different contributors but we would not wish it to be regarded as a collection of entirely separate essays. Many of the ideas, which have grown out of our interest in and enthusiasm for an aspect of social work which has a central place in the work of almost all social workers, have been discussed and developed during the several years that we have worked together at the University College of North Wales. We each have our own preferences and emphasis but it would be hard for any one of us to lay special claim to particular ideas.

We are indebted to those colleagues in the Department of Social Theory and Institutions at Bangor who have listened patiently, as well as to those students who have helped us to clarify our thoughts and to progress. Our thanks are also due to Sally Pritchard, Kath Thomas, and Pat Ormond for their help with typing. We would like particularly to thank Tom Douglas for his support and guidance.

Part One

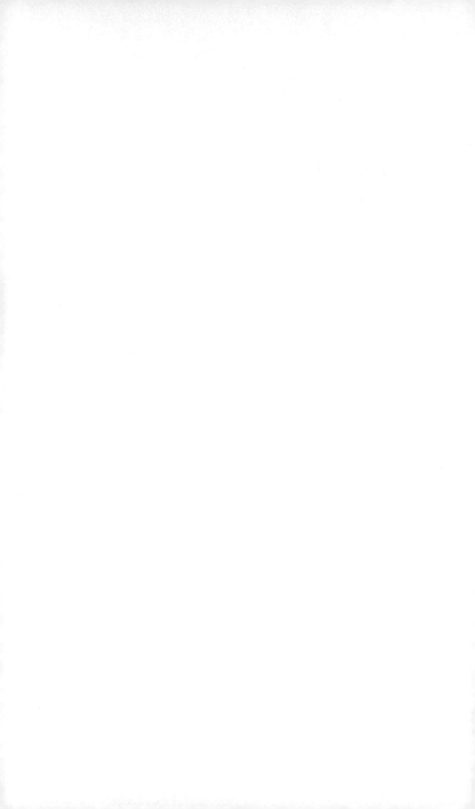

Introduction   *Paul Brearley*

In an activity as diffuse as social work it is inevitable that some words and phrases will appear more frequently than others in the mass of writing and be used as pegs on which to hang groups of thoughts and ideas. Some of the language of social work is obscure, and overworked, and some has deteriorated sadly into jargon – graphically defined by the Oxford Dictionary as the 'twittering of birds'. It is not the aim of this book to add one more attempt to the many efforts to define the nature, or essential elements of social work. Some of the words and expressions that social workers use have, however, an immediacy and relevance to the everyday task. One word that does stand out, if only because of the frequency with which it is used, is *care*.

Caring is a feeling that is experienced by people and is also something that is done by some people for others. The concept of care has been used widely in many different ways and in many different contexts. There can be few activities in which social workers are involved more frequently than admission to care. The phrase 'admission to care' will call up vivid memories for almost every social worker. To admit someone to care is often to be involved in a major life change for an individual and for those around him, usually at a time of distress, and crisis. The events that happen during admission to care can be magnified for everyone involved and the things that are done to, and with, and around a client at this time often have a lasting effect.

Admitting people to care is a frequent activity for most social workers and yet, although there have been a number of small pamphlets, and many journal articles, it is a subject that has never been written about at length. It is the aim of this book to explore some of the elements of the process of admission to care in the light of the statutory duties and responsibilities of social workers, and in relation to the hazards and dangers to which both social workers and clients are exposed.

RESOURCES FOR CARING

There are differences between those forms of care which are concerned to provide treatment or rehabilitation, those which contain or restrict, and those which are mainly concerned with supporting and providing a safe living environment. It is arguable that most admissions involve a mixture of at least two of these aims. The possibility of conflict and confusion of aims and purposes exists in all admissions and the social worker has a responsibility to clarify these aims as far as possible. This is particularly so when resources are both scarce and expensive.

Historically the practice of paying people to care has had a patchy development but there can be no doubt that the resources of institutions and foster care are now very extensive and very costly. In 1977, for instance, there were over 101,000 children in care in England and Wales, as compared to a figure of 62,200 in 1961. Of those in care in 1977 just over 40,000 were in some form of institutional accommodation and a further 36,000 were in hostels, lodgings, or were boarded out. In 1976 there were over 6,000 physically disabled people under 65 years of age in local authority residential homes, and a further 6,000 were in private or voluntary homes. Over 11,000 mentally handicapped people under 65, in England and Wales, were in some form of residential accommodation in 1977.

Among the elderly 3 per cent of men and 5 per cent of women over the age of 65 are in residential institutions – old people's homes, or hospitals – and among the over 85s the proportions increase to 13 per cent of men and 19 per cent of woman. In psychiatric hospitals the average daily occupancy of mental illness beds in 1977 was 105,000 (Central Statistical Office 1979). Clearly large numbers of people experience institutional care, and other forms of organized caring.

CONTINUUM OF CARE

The expression 'a continuum of care' is one that has had wide usage in recent years. A continuum refers to an unbroken course of events and the most common inference to be drawn from the use of the expression is that caring resources are in a continuous and interchangeable relationship to each other. The individual client is expected to be able to move within the range of caring resources and to be at the right place, at the right time for his* own needs. In one sense the caring continuum might be regarded as a linear conception with the client beginning at one end and growing or living through the experience of change of living environments until he emerges at the other end. The client, for instance, might be seen in this sense as leaving an unsuitable home environment to live in a Children's Home, then with foster parents, before finally growing to independent adult status. From another perspective the caring continuum may be be seen as a circular experience as, for example, when admission to a psychiatric hospital is arranged from the patient's home, and after treatment the patient returns to the same home with, perhaps, day hospital attendance before full independence.

An underlying assumption of this view of the caring system as a set of interchangeable options, in which the client chooses, or is helped to choose the most suitable resource for his needs, is that choice exists. Plank (1977), writing about the elderly, has argued that such a view is unrealistic and suggests that since options are not available it is nonsense to think that elderly clients can be helped to make choices between residential care, sheltered housing, and domiciliary care. Similar arguments might be advanced about child care: when foster parents are scarce it is unrealistic to think in terms of ideal placements, and the question is more often what is possible than what is desirable.

In a discussion of residential care David Ennals (1978)

* Where the sex of social worker or client is not defined by the particular circumstances described, he or she is referred to, for convenience, in the masculine gender throughout this book; such references should be taken to imply male or female.

accepts that residential care is not necessarily the best or most appropriate way of meeting a particular individual's needs: 'it is simply the best that is available, the most expedient.' He does, however, acknowledge that residential care can be, in an absolute sense, the best that can be done. To admit someone to care may be inevitable and expedient, in the sense that there is little choice available at the time but it may also be the appropriate action for the client. All too often residential resources in particular have been described in gloomy terms but it is possible to evolve ways of using caring resources in a more flexible way.

As Utting (1977) has said, 'the problem is to determine what the right things are for residential care to do: and then for residential care to do them well'. Similarly if admission to care is either inevitable or desirable (or both) then good standards of practice in the admission situation should be identified and developed.

One important aspect of the better use of caring resources is the relationship between different groups of workers in each setting. A working party report of the Central Council for Education and Training in Social Work (1973) has emphasized that residential care is an intrinsic part of social work, although recognizing that it has specialized knowledge and skills in addition to the basic elements of social work. All the work of residential centres is not necessarily social work, however. A more recent BASW working party report (BASW 1977a) points out, for instance, that those skills which are concerned with creating physical care and a safe environment are not necessarily social work tasks, although they may be integral to social work within a residential setting. The differences and relationships between field workers and residential workers are of central importance to some, though not all, forms of admission. In the case of admission to psychiatric hospital, or of admission to geriatric or children's hospitals, the issues are different but equally complex. The links between the social work and medical professions are intricate and not always amicable. Whether admission to care involves the client in moving to live with foster parents, to residential care, or to hospital it is essential that good working relationships exist if the client is to benefit from the available options.

VULNERABILITY AND ADMISSION

Payne (1977), reporting discussions with residential workers, says that they refer, above all, to their sense of isolation, their lack of professional identity, and feelings that their contribution is insufficiently valued. Dunham (1978) identifies reorganization and other changes, role conflict and role uncertainty, poor working conditions, and communication difficulties as major stress situations for residential workers. Jones (1976), discussing social work in broader terms, examines the extent to which social workers have a duty to care and whether a breach of such a duty could lead to a court action for neglect.

The vulnerability and stress of social workers in other words has become a major preoccupation in recent years. To a large extent this is a direct consequence of the spate of enquiries into cases of child abuse. Social workers are concerned with their own self protection and in situations where they are faced with emotional or physical as well as legal risks this is hardly surprising. One danger of this trend is that the needs of clients may take second place although, since the social workers' principal security lies in good practice, this need not be the case.

The risks to the social worker and to the client, in terms of recognizable hazards and dangers, are a central feature of admission to care and will be dealt with centrally in this book.

The book is, then, concerned with the discussion of two central concepts in social work. In the first place there is a detailed examination of one kind of major life transition: admission to care. This will be linked with an elaboration of the concept of risk which is a central element in social work decision making. The existing literature relating to both risk, and to the admission transition is widely scattered and has never been brought together in comprehensive form. The importance of bringing these ideas together rests directly on the fact that social workers — whether in the field or in residential care — are continuously engaged in the admission of clients to care as well as in the analysis and management of risk factors. The discussion that follows will consider risk, and admission, and the legal framework of admission. This discussion forms the basis of the later chapters which will identify the specific problems of good practice in admitting different groups of clients to care. Finally there is a discussion of alternatives to residential care with regard to the specific example of the elderly: Glenys Jones demonstrates that residential care is not the only way of caring for old people and neither is it necessarily the last resort – for some people it may be the best solution chosen realistically from a range of options.

1 A Preliminary Framework for Risk Analysis *Paul Brearley*

The concept of risk has appeared more and more frequently in recent social work writing and even in terms of the most simple use of the expression it is obvious that risk plays a very important part in the work of social workers. People of all ages go into a variety of different forms of care because they are exposed to an equally wide variety of risks: it is recognized that there are a number of undesirable possibilities in their current life situations. In this sense residential care, as well as other kinds of care which will be considered in Chapter 8, aims to offer an environment which has reduced, or even eliminated some of these risks.

Yet this simplistic presentation of the function of residential care is itself dangerous. There is ample evidence that the actual process of moving from one place to another, of leaving behind a familiar environment, and of entering a strange, unfamiliar environment carries with it a new set of risks − both physical and emotional. Similarly, life in an enclosed institutional situation involves exposure to a further set of risks which have been well described and documented.

Clearly risk is an important aspect of admission to care − before, during, and after the move from one place to another − yet there have been no detailed attempts to define or analyse the underlying meanings of the term. One short recent work suggests that 'the question of risk in social work has been increasingly on people's minds in recent times' and proceeds to emphasize the importance of identifying 'potential risk situations' (National Association of Probation Officers 1977:5). It is certainly not clear from much of the literature how a risk situation is to be identified and this seems to be such a major feature of social work practice in the context of admission to residential care that the basic elements of the risk concept will be explored here before the discussion moves on to consider the actual process of admission.

The term 'risk' is used in a variety of ways within the social work literature. This variation can be illustrated by a brief consideration of some recent work. The *at-risk* concept, for example, is in common usage in social work, particularly in relation to children. The BASW document, 'The Social Work Task', in discussing criteria for deciding whether the skills of a professionally qualified social worker are required seems to equate at-riskness with vulnerability: 'The typical example of clients with high physical vulnerability is children at-risk of non-accidental injury' (BASW 1977a:43). The same document continues to discuss 'the risk of delinquency, mental illness and social disfunctioning', also under the heading of *vulnerability*.

At-riskness is not of course confined to children and a recent study of hypothermia among the elderly makes frequent use of the concept (Wicks 1978). This study suggests that one tenth of the elderly sample were 'at risk' of their inner body temperature falling to a level that, it is commonly accepted, constitutes hypothermia. In this context the term appears to imply that certain people were *more likely* than others to experience the undesirable outcome of hypothermia. The study also discusses various social factors which may be associated with the likelihood of hypothermia.

The possibility of identifying those features of situations which are associated with undesirable outcome – or which might be regarded as predictors of certain outcomes – has been a preoccupation of many other researchers and writers. One recent study by NSPCC workers (NSPCC 1976:210) of at-risk situations involving children illustrates this. In concluding, the authors comment that 'findings suggest a multi-causal model . . . certain factors do seem to be more prevalent than others . . . factors include the fragmented and emotionally demanding childhoods of many abusive parents, the fact that most of our study children were unwanted at the

time of birth, marital disharmony, overcrowded and inadequate accommodation, social isolation and rootlessness.'

Even such brief illustrations begin to bring out some of the
component parts. At-riskness is a commonly used concept
which involves vulnerability to loss or damage, an element of
likelihood or probability, and the possibility of discovering
associated factors and predictors of greater likelihood.

To be at risk is usually presented as an undesirable condition.
A seminar report, for instance, quotes the admissions procedure to Old People's Homes in use in Coventry Social
Services Department – 'highest priority grade (is) accorded
where there is a high and continuing risk factor in the social
situation despite the maximum possible input of fieldwork and
domiciliary services' (DHSS 1976a). Risk is, therefore, the
cause of admission to care and yet the Personal Social Service
Council are able to recommend, when discussing standards of
practice in residential care for adults that 'Acceptance of risk is
fundamental to good residential care, both for the resident and
for the staff' (PSSC 1977 : para. 1.17). Each of these apparently
contradictory positions has a separate credibility and their
contradiction – that risk is a reason for care but also a desirable
feature of subsequent care – stems partly from the problem of
definition. A further examination of the PSSC document gives
some clarification:

> 'there is considerable tension between ensuring the safety yet
> promoting the freedom of people in care, between offering
> protection yet providing a convenient and reasonably low-
> cost environment, and between avoiding the visible instance
> of harm on the one hand and the promotion of a high quality
> of everyday life for residents on the other. Inevitably some
> risks do have to be taken' (para. 1.16).

A feature of this use of the term risk is the balancing of freedom
with safety. It is also suggested that 'all residents should have
the right . . . to take risks and be responsible for their own
behaviour, where this does not reduce the quality of life, or
safety of others' (para. 2.7). Risk, then, has a linked concept –
responsibility – which is in turn linked to choice: 'Residents

cannot live full and interesting lives, if all choice or responsibility is removed from them' (para. 4.2). This use of risk seems to be concerned with allowing freedom of choice – the right to make decisions which involve possible danger and therefore to *take risks*.

A major distinction to be found in social work thinking, then, is between the concepts of at-riskness and risk-taking. These will be examined further in the light of more detailed definitions.

RISK: SOME TERMS DEFINED

The NAPO booklet on risk referred to earlier (NAPO 1977) chooses to quote a basic dictionary definition and suggests that '"risk" may be simply defined as "danger; peril; hazard; the chance of bad consequences; or the amount covered by insurance".' This approach embodies two components which are both of obvious importance in practice. The first of these is the negative outcome implied in the earlier discussion in terms of physical, psychological, or social damage. The second is the element of uncertainty that a particular outcome will come about. These two elements, which for the time being can be called *damage* and *chance* are closely linked in many ways and seem to become unhelpfully tangled in the social work literature. How helpful is it, for instance, to talk of a risky situation? This may mean that the situation is simply unclear, or uncertain, or that negative outcomes may result but it gives little clue to the analysis of the relative likelihood of certain outcomes, or of the relative importance of possible outcomes. If a child is at-risk that is clearly important but more information is necessary: what are the possible losses in the situation?; how likely is it that each one will come about?; what can be done to avoid some outcomes, or to minimize their likelihood?

A good deal of thinking about the nature of risk has taken place in the commercial insurance field and some useful contributions to definition can be added from that source. Greene (1977) defines risk as uncertainty as to loss, and distinguishes between objective risk on the one hand, as the relative variation of actual from probable loss, and subjective risk on the other hand. Subjective risk refers to the mental state of an individual who experiences uncertainty, doubt, or worry as to the outcome of a given event.

A further definition is made between pure risk which exists when there is uncertainty as to whether the destruction of an object will occur, and speculative risk when there is uncertainty about an event under consideration that could produce either a profit or a loss. This distinction highlights the important difference between the undesirable risk situation in which there is a possibility of loss or damage and the risk-taking situation in which something is put at stake in the anticipation of possible future gain.

Three basic definitions can therefore be offered on which to build further analysis.

(1) *Risk* refers to uncertainty as to loss. Any situation in which there is a possibility of loss, whatever the degree of probability that the outcome will or will not occur, is a risky situation.

(2) A *danger* is a contingency which, if it occurs, may cause loss, damage, or diminution.

(3) A *hazard* is defined as a condition which introduces the possibility and increases the probability that loss, damage, or diminution will result from danger.

It is important to recognize that what is being proposed in these definitions is a differentiation between uncertainty and probability. Social workers are arguably always concerned with uncertainty and whilst not necessarily a constant factor this is a given element in all action (in the sense that all life situations are uncertain) and assessment. On the other hand social workers are constantly concerned with evaluating and balancing the likelihood of certain events occurring against the probable effect of possible courses of action. Risk as uncertainty, then, is a given factor in situations and requires particular techniques of management whereas likelihood can be assessed, evaluated, and balanced in action decisions and requires different techniques of management. Some helpful attempts have already been made in work with suspected child injury situations to classify probability. NSPCC registers, for instance, use a five-point Index of Suspicion ranging from 'certain' through 'very suspicious', 'suspicious', and 'accidental' to 'prodromal' (Creighton and Outram 1977).

In the framework of the basic definitions it is possible to confirm the difference between two of the concepts identified in the social work literature and to add a third in the action setting.

(1) *At-riskness* is the passive component of the social work perspective, in which at least one potential negative outcome exists and is identified in the status quo. Expressed differently, at-riskness implies that the client is exposed to hazards which may create recognizable danger.

(2) *Risk-taking behaviour* occurs when the actor recognizes that he is irreversibly exposed to a potential negative outcome in following a course of action which may also lead to a potential positive outcome. In taking a risk the actor consciously puts something at stake in the hope of reaching a desired goal.

(3) *Risky actions* are those actions in which the outcomes are uncertain and at least one of the potential outcomes is regarded as negative. It is worth pointing out in this context that social workers may talk about selecting the course of action of greatest potential gain but in many cases they are as likely to be concerned with the course of action of least potential loss.

The definitions can be extended in one final respect: the differentiation that is being made is intended to contribute to both risk-analysis and risk-management, and offers a framework for decision making. Within the framework different aspects of choice can be highlighted.

(1) *Choice*: a decision between alternatives.
(2) *Risky Choice*: a decision in which the actor will be exposed to uncertain outcomes at least one of which is potentially negative. The social worker will take decisions which expose

both himself and his clients to uncertain outcomes and he is therefore involved in *bearing risks* himself and in *allocating risks* to others.

(3) *Choice dilemma*: a decision between at least two courses of action, the possible outcomes of which are likely to be unfavourable.

The most important of these definitions are those which distinguish uncertainty from probability: risk is simply uncertainty as to loss; danger is that which may occur and cause loss; and a hazard is an existing factor which makes loss from the danger possible or more likely. The clearest illustration of these distinctions can be found in the insurance field. Driving a car is risky in that there is always a chance of negative outcomes: the probability of each outcome can be statistically calculated and an insurance value attached to it. One danger in driving the car is that there will be a collision which may result in specific losses, some of which are more likely than others. Driving the car on a wet road, or at speed around a corner is hazardous because these factors increase the likelihood of the collision.

In a social work context isolation is a hazard to loneliness, the unwanted pregnancy is a hazard to child battering, and unemployment is a hazard to poverty.

If these concepts can be clarified and separated out then a framework for analysis and action in the risky situation (i.e. in which at least one danger is recognized) is possible.

A RISK-ANALYSIS FRAMEWORK

It has already been suggested that social workers are inevitably dealing with uncertainties and that they are as likely to be concerned with minimizing loss as with maximizing gain. When the dangers, hazards, strengths, and potential gains and losses are identified the worker and client engage in a balancing operation, which is rarely static, and usually involves a series of rebalancing and reassessing operations. The modification of assessment through action is, of course, entirely familiar to the social worker but the balancing of probabilities and uncertainties involves four underlying considerations through-out the analysis/action process.

(1) *Awareness of potential outcomes*: this will involve the level of knowledge and information available about the possible outcomes of action, or non-action.
(2) *Certainty or likelihood of potential outcomes*: when possible outcomes have been recognized it is necessary to consider the relative likelihood that each will occur.
(3) The *ascribed gravity or importance of potential outcomes*: the relative importance of each outcome to the social worker, and to the client, in the light of what is known about the likelihood of each is an essential calculation. Through this element possible outcomes are given a value and come to be regarded as potential gains, or potential losses. This can be termed the utility of the outcome.
(4) The *imminence of the consequences* and the overall time dimension is of major importance. The imminence of the danger is what is likely to turn a difficult problem into an emergency.

With these factors in mind – and also bearing in mind the importance of prevailing decision-rules in risky situations – the risk/danger/hazard distinction can be applied to case situations.

The Case of Mrs K

Aged 82, widowed seven years, a son living in America and a daughter, herself 63, living about seven miles away. For several years she has suffered from angina with heart failure. On two occasions she has been taken ill in the street but has returned home by taxi, refusing to allow an ambulance to be called, or to tell the doctor, although she is receiving tablets.

She lives alone and discourages contact with the neighbours who are willing and able to help but have several times been rebuffed. The daughter visits three times a week but has to come by bus. She is herself unwell, and her husband, who has recently retired, resents her giving so much time. Apart from the daughter's visits Mrs K has contact with the home help, the milkman, and bread delivery man. She goes to the shops twice each week but is unsteady when walking and finds the walk distressing. The house is small and she sleeps downstairs but there are two steps from the living-room to the kitchen and an open fire for which she refuses to use a guard.

In recent months she has become very forgetful and a little confused and has twice burned out kettles on the gas stove. A social worker visited to discuss admission to residential care but on the fourth visit Mrs K refused to allow her in the house.

The first step in analysis is to identify the general hazards: what are the factors in the situation which introduce the likelihood of an undesirable occurrence. These can be listed as predictive hazards. In Mrs K's case a number of features can be said to increase the statistical probability of negative outcome. People over the age of 75, for instance, are more vulnerable to physical danger, to loneliness, and are more likely to be in poor health (see, for example, Abrams 1978). Similarly isolation predisposes to a subjective feeling of loneliness which in turn may lead to other negatives.

The second step is to list those hazards which exist in the situation and which may precipitate specific dangers (i.e. increase the likelihood of a loss outcome). An unguarded fire, for example, has specific possible outcomes – particularly fire, or burns. Similarly, although angina is treatable it predisposes to physical dangers which may be precipitated in the form of a severe or fatal attack as a result of failure to seek or follow treatment.

Third, the dangers begin to emerge in association with these hazards. If the feared contingencies can be identified then they can be weighed in terms of the factors suggested – information, likelihood of outcome, relative value, and imminence.

If this procedure is followed in relation to each of the actors involved, a second balancing operation can be undertaken in terms of the focus to be taken: a decision on priorities is made. In this case, for instance, the social worker may choose to value the possible blame that may be attached to herself, or the guilt she would feel on Mrs K's death, more highly than the loss of rights which Mrs K would experience if she is not given the opportunity to express her own wishes. Similarly the dangers to Mrs K must be assessed in relation to the dangers to her daughter who may have to continue to carry a heavy burden of work and responsibility.

This can be outlined schematically (see *Table 1(1)*). The lists are illustrative, and not comprehensive: and an important component – the existing strengths of the situation – is omitted at this stage to simplify the discussion.

TABLE 1(1)

	Predictive hazards	*Situational hazards*	*Dangers*

Mrs K	Age
	Widowed
	Poor health
	Few relatives
	Mental frailty
		Isolation/lack
		  of support
		Withdrawal/
		  rejecting
		  behaviour
		Steps to
		  kitchen/
		  unsteady on
		  her feet
		Fire/no guard
		Gas cooker/
		  forgetfulness
		Angina/
		  reluctance to
		  seek treatment
		Growing
		  confusion
			Loneliness
			Fall
			Fire/burn
			Heart attack
			Lack of
			  attention to
			  her wishes
			Admission to
			  care

Daughter	Poor health
	Increasing age
	  etc. of Mrs K
		Husband's
		  demands
		Increasing needs
		  of Mrs K
		Frequent
		  travelling
			Death of Mrs K
			Increasing
			  demands of
			  Mrs K
			Marital stress
			Breakdown of
			  health

TABLE 1(1)—cont.

	Predictive hazards	Situational hazards	Dangers
Son-in-law	Increasing age, etc. of Mrs K Wife's poor health	Wife's health/ travelling Increasing needs of Mrs K	Death of Mrs K Increasing demands of Mrs K on wife Marital stress
Neighbours	Increasing age, etc. of Mrs K	Increasing needs of Mrs K	Increasing demand for care from Mrs K Fire
Social Worker	Mrs K's attitude to others Available resources Lack of resources		Death of Mrs K Criticism of neighbours/ daughter/or others Leaving Mrs K at home without adequate resources
	Attitudes of community etc. to the 'elderly at risk'	Failure to establish adequate relationships	Admitting Mrs K to res. care (and guilt if should not respond favourably to the move, or even die)

The strengths of this form of analysis are considerable. In the first place it offers a clear outline of key factors and their relationship to each other for each of the actors in the situation. Second, it identifies the dangers − those contingencies which must be avoided if loss, damage, or other diminution are to be averted − and these dangers can be given a relative value: it offers a framework for priority decisions. Third, it highlights the relationship between the dangers and those factors which make it likely that loss will result and it therefore becomes possible to evaluate the probability of *counter-balancing* the hazards. If the precipitative hazards can be offset, even in the light of the predictors, it will be possible to reduce the likelihood of danger, or to 'minimize the risk'.

In Mrs K's situation the dangers to the old lady are clearly pressing but some of these will require more urgent attention than others. The physical dangers which might occur – she may have a heart attack, or a fall, or burn herself, or leave the gas cooker on and cause a fire – are likely to cause damage to Mrs K or her property which will be very difficult to repair. These dangers are also imminent in the sense that they might occur at any time whereas others – loneliness, stress, or failure to respect her wishes – are longer-term events. The physical dangers are therefore not necessarily more important but they are more urgent and require early action. They are more likely, more imminent, and represent a high risk.

Once the dangers have been arranged in priority order the analysis points to action possibilities. If the danger of fire is made likely by the lack of a fire-guard or lack of modification to the cooker then the reduction in probability of fire is fairly simple. If, on the other hand, the danger of fire is introduced because of her increasing mental confusion and is increased by her inability to cope with the cooker or to remember to put the fire-guard up the solutions may be more complex but can be equally clearly identified.

So far, the framework for analysis has offered what is effectively a modified and extended 'problem list' approach. A further element can be added to extend the concept of balancing of uncertainties with available action options. It is important to identify the strengths, as well as the weaknesses in each situation.

The D Family

Mr and Mrs D married when she was 18 and he was 20. At the time of the marriage she was six months pregnant. Mr D is not the father of the child, a boy who is now 6 years old. There is a second son of the marriage who is 4 years old.

Their daughter, Tracy, was born 18 months ago and at the age of 7 months she was taken to the hospital casualty department with a suspected broken arm. Mrs D said she had fallen from her pram and after she was found to have old fractures of both tibiae a Place of Safety order was taken and later a Care Order was made, but opposed by Mr and Mrs D.

Suitable foster parents could not be found and Tracy has been in a Residential Nursery since that time. Mrs D has been encouraged to visit her there but has found the visits distressing and now rarely goes to see Tracy. This has antagonized the Nursery Staff.

Mr D's own father died when he was a baby and he is very close to his mother who is diabetic and unable to give any real help. Several months ago he returned to live with her for two weeks following an argument with his wife. Mrs D is closely involved with her mother and sister who both live nearby and they tend to encourage her in frequent rows with Mr D who they do not like. Mrs D's mother often looks after the two boys.

They have recently been rehoused from a small maisonette to a three-bedroomed council house. Mr D is unemployed and Mrs D has not worked since they married and before that time her work record was uneven. A social worker is visiting regularly.

They have asked that Tracy should be returned home. Mrs D is now three months pregnant.

The information given in this case is very limited and in no way adequate to a decision — indeed the obvious decision is to seek more information. Nevertheless it is sufficient to illustrate the method of analysis.

Once again the stages are clear.

(1) Identify the predictors in the light of information about the probability of loss or damage in similar situations.
(2) Identify the specific factors which increase the likelihood of a loss outcome.
(3) Identify the strengths — those factors which may reduce the likelihood of a loss. This is the final element to be weighed in the balance when identifying the dangers.
(4) Identify the dangers.

In reality it is unlikely that these stages will follow neatly one from another but it is essential to clarify the relationship of each set of factors in the situation to the anticipated or potential outcomes.

In the case of the D family analysis of Tracy's current position reveals several factors (the list in *Table 1(2a)* is illustrative, not complete).

TABLE 1(2a)

	Predictive hazards	Situational hazards	Strengths	Dangers
Tracy (if not returned)	Separation from parents	No foster parents available Mothers irregular visiting Attitude of Nursery Staff	Physical safety Social Worker Concern of Nursery Staff	Psychological/ emotional damage if: i) Remain in nursery ii) Return home Rejection

A further analysis of one potential course of action — Tracy's return home — involves a different range of factors (once again *Table 1(2b)* is an incomplete but illustrative list).

TABLE 1(2b)

	Predictive hazards	Situational hazards	Strengths	Dangers
Tracy (if returned)	Parents early, 'shotgun' marriage Father's own parenting experience Mother's own parenting experience	Unemploy- ment Mrs D's pregnancy Marital stress Mrs D's mother's attitude to marital stress	Mrs D's mothers willingness Rehoused No indica- tion that brothers have been abused	Physical abuse Psychological/ emotional damage

TABLE 1(2b)—cont.

Predictive hazards	Situational hazards	Strengths	Dangers
	Separation from parents for almost one year and spasmodic contact	Social Worker	

The categorization of these factors requires very careful consideration. The fact that Mrs D's mother is able to help with the children may, in fact, be a hazard not a strength if her own skills are inadequate. The placing of each factor in any one category therefore involves careful and detailed information collection and handling. Nevertheless it becomes plain that the relevance of each factor is likely to vary depending on the course of action, or non-action, that is proposed. The decision on Tracy's future rests on the relative importance or likelihood of each identified danger. It depends also on the estimates made of the possibilities and probabilities of offsetting each hazard and on the anticipated likelihood that the strengths available will balance out the hazards. Two questions are important.

(1) Can uncertainty be tolerated in the light of the possible outcome: if there is any chance of physical damage can a risk be taken?
(2) If uncertainty can be permitted what is the degree of probability of negative outcome beyond which the risk is unacceptable?

So far it has been assumed that the dangers to Tracy are of paramount importance and in this case it would be difficult, in the climate of present opinion, to dispute this. It is not necessarily easy, however, to rank the dangers to other participants in this situation in priority order. Some of the dangers of returning Tracy home can be listed: space does not permit a full analysis but some of the more obvious dangers are given in *Table 1(2c)*.

TABLE 1(2c)

	Dangers
Tracy	Physical abuse (death)
	Psychological/emotional damage
Mr and Mrs D	Physical/emotional stress
	Physical abuse of Tracy
	Guilt
	Prosecution
	Marital stress/separation
Brothers	Parents separation/divorce
	Physical abuse (death)
	Psychological/emotional damage
Unborn child	Miscarriage
	Physical abuse following birth (death)
Social Worker	Abuse of Tracy (death)
	Blame/enquiry
	Guilt

Clearly the dangers to Tracy are the primary consideration here but the relative weighting of other dangers is not so easy. If she were returned home, should the worker focus on Mrs D and the unborn child, or on the marital relationship, or on the dangers to the two brothers and the possibility of using their grandmother to contribute to their care? The answers are, of course, to be found in the relative likelihoods and value of each course of action and its anticipated outcome.

To summarize the outline framework for risk analysis, it is being suggested that all social work situations involve uncertainty. It is possible to clarify and organize factors within a situation through the defined concepts of hazard (precipitating and situationally specific), strength, and danger. These will be ascribed relevance and value in relation to anticipated, potential, or likely outcomes which may be identified as potential losses, or potential gains. The concept of risk itself is neutral but at-riskness and risk-taking have important value components which must be identified, balanced, and counter-balanced in action. Balancing and counterbalancing is a continuous process which takes account of what is known about outcomes, their likelihood, gravity, and imminence. Particularly important is the probability that an outcome will occur: in other words, what is known or believed about possible outcomes. The likely loss outcome of a particular situation may become the hazard to a further danger in the subsequent context. Similarly the potential gain may become one of the strengths of the subsequent situation. For instance, a potential gain of leaving Tracy in the nursery is the possibility of gaining a foster-placement for her. This would then become a strength as a firm base for building Tracy's future in later action.

Within social work thinking there has been a particular emphasis on the problem: problem definition, problem explanation, problem solving, etc. have played a major part in social work assessment and action. Attempts have been made to discuss the problem-solving process in some detail (see, for example, Pincus and Minahan 1973). These attempts have suggested that the process involves, for example, information collection, ascribing relevance to information, goal setting, decision making, action, learning, and evaluation. The process element appears prominently (see Whittaker 1974) in other aspects of social work in the recognition that growth and change involves transition; from, for example, one social status to another, or from one life stage to another. Sometimes transitions are seen as positive (marriage, graduation), or neutral, and sometimes as negative (retirement, bereavement). The process view of human development, or of forms of social work action, such as admission to care is difficult to reconcile with the problem-solving focus of much social work action. This difficulty can be stated simplistically as the difference between the problem, as a static concept, defined as a doubtful or difficult issue, and the process as a changing course through time.

It is suggested that the form of analysis offered here gives an action framework for both the understanding of social work situations, and the identification of courses of action in relation to the outcome potentials, which in turn point to further action possibilities. The problem solution has a change potential in so far as actors in the situation are able to anticipate and value action/non-action options in terms of their likely outcomes. A criticism that has been made of the social systems theory approach to providing a unified model for social work practice has been that it does not make sufficient accommodation to the uncertainty of human values and affairs. The theories currently being developed gloss over, it is suggested, the ethical dilemmas and hard choices between conflicting priorities which are central to practitioners work (Davies and McLeod 1978). The risk-analysis framework offers a way of overcoming this within three everyday concepts – hazards, strengths, and dangers.

What is offered at this point is an outline structure for thinking which appears to have room within it for many theoretical, or ideological stances. In individual or generalized situations a causal model can be constructed within the framework and the model becomes active through its predictive components and through its ability to change through action and modification within the basic headings. Factors in each case may be ascribed significance for understanding, prescription, or action on the basis of one or more models or theories. It would, for instance, be quite possible to analyse a situation in social systems theory terms within the risk-analysis framework. In a given situation the hazards and strengths which exist may introduce, increase, or decrease dangers and affect the loss/gain possibilities for various social systems – client, target, change agent, etc. (Pincus and Minahan 1973). On the other hand the theoretical stance taken may alter the significance, or ascribed importance of existing factors or anticipated outcomes. The importance and relevance of separation from her parents for Tracy D for social work action is clearly different from a psychodynamic than from a learning theory perspective.

Such a structure for thinking and describing situations is, of course, only useful in so far as it helps the social worker define and follow through a course of action. In the following chapter consideration will be given to acting in risky situations: to the management of hazards and the understanding of dangers.

2 Managing Risk and Taking Action *Paul Brearley*

A number of writers have discussed or outlined areas of thinking that relate to the management of risk, danger, or uncertainty. Golan, for instance, in an early discussion of crisis theory considered crisis intervention in apparently similar terms to those that are being used in the present discussion. She outlines the hazardous event, the vulnerable state, the precipitating factor, and the state of active crisis (Golan 1969). Although similar in some respects to the ideas discussed here the concept of the state of active crisis − 'the stage of disequilibrium, when tension and anxiety have risen to a peak and the individual's homeostatic devices no longer operate' − is largely a descriptive device. The relationship of the crisis state to other elements in the development of the process of change is primarily in terms of phases of change through time. The relationship between the causes of change and the action potential is less important, within the crisis theory framework, than the potential of the actual crisis situation for change. In the crisis state, in terms of the risk analysis framework, elements of the situation are identifiable as hazardous in that they are likely to contribute to dangerous outcomes which can be specified. These hazards will have an action context in so far as they can or cannot be removed, altered, or diminished. Risk analysis is an additional tool which can be applied in the crisis intervention context, as in other theoretical contexts. It suggests that factors in a situation must be clearly identified and that they have relevance to the social worker in terms of their relationship to other factors and to possible actions and outcomes.

Bloom (1975) has undertaken a much more detailed analysis

of some of the concepts involved in this discussion but uses a rather different basic framework. He distinguishes between theory, strategy, and action. Whichever theory is chosen, he suggests, a further issue arises in relation to the translation of that theory into a form that can be used by the helping professional. This translation of theory into practice results through strategy, and he makes the very important point that strategies are highly saturated with values. Bloom also discusses some other important elements which have only been alluded to here. The issues of how individuals acquire and use concepts, and social constructs; of how research findings can be used to identify predictive hazards, or potential action outcomes; and of possible approaches to information collection, are all directly relevant to the use of the risk analysis framework. Each of these, and many other elements require much more detailed examination if all the other implications of this approach are to be fully understood.

The most helpful contribution of Bloom's work to the present discussion lies in his consideration of how inferences about outcome are to be made. The risk analysis framework requires the worker to possess or develop skills of anticipation. This implies that workers should be able to carry out two processes:

(1) identify what is possible: to understand the range of actions and outcomes is essential;
(2) to consider how likely outcomes are.

Bloom suggests two methods of inferring outcomes, and thereby of bridging theory and practice: the deductive model, relying largely on existing concepts and knowledge, and the inductive which starts with events and proceeds pragmatically. This bridge of theory to practice has specific relevance to social work situations in its recognition of probability and is a central part of risk analysis. Bloom is more concerned, however, with the improvement of techniques of measurement to *increase* the workers ability to recognize probability of outcome. It seems likely that social workers will always be working in situations of uncertainty and the contribution of the risk analysis framework is rather to *structure* knowledge about the existing probability of outcome.

Even the most tentative steps into risk analysis reveal the complexity of issues and demands. The framework does not exclude existing theories and approaches but differs from most of these in its focus on the action component against the background of probability and uncertainty. Conceptualizations about social work have most frequently taken separate emphases on fragments of the total picture: the theory – strategy – action division is a partialization just as much as the groupwork – casework – community work division. If knowledge of factors in the situation (hazards and strengths) can be interrelated with anticipations of outcomes of various action/non-action possibilities in a clear structure the totality of any situation emerges. This does, however, pose new questions for social work knowledge and skills. Within risk-analysis a greater emphasis is placed on the worker's ability to anticipate and it therefore becomes important to understand the meaning and nature of anticipation. It has already been suggested that anticipating implies being able to identify what is possible and what is likely. To a large extent this simply means the use of familiar skills of information collection, decision making etc., but it will also involve a consideration of the important part played by subjective and experiential factors in the formation of constructs for the individual and for the social group. The use of constructed assumptions by the social worker in deducing, or inducing potential outcomes is an important but neglected area in social work training. There is, of course, also a close link between these issues and decision-making theory.

The risk-analysis framework is firstly a structure for the organization of knowledge for action in specific situations. It is an additional tool which can be operated in conjunction with widely differing explanatory models and theories and rests partly on the assumption that an organized approach to action and goal-setting are helpful to the social worker. In the sense that it accommodates both uncertainty and probability the framework seems useful for all social work situations. It has, in other words, a general application. It is, however, possible to define certain situations encountered by social workers more precisely as both uncertain − risky − and *dangerous* in that the potential outcomes are:

(1) demonstrably highly probable in the light of the existing hazards and strengths; and/or
(2) demonstrably highly undesirable in the context of prevailing social values.

It is this feature of risk which underlies the recurring concept of at-riskness discussed earlier. In these terms the child at-risk is the child who can be shown to be exposed to recognizable hazards which introduce and increase the likelihood of physical and emotional damage. At the present time public reaction to highly publicized child deaths (see, for example, DHSS 1974) has led to an emphasis on physical safety in particular. Other particularly dangerous situations in social work relate to the elderly at-risk who are exposed to dangers of illness, hypothermia, malnutrition, etc.; the mentally ill who are exposed to the dangers of self-damage, or of damaging others, or of loss of liberty, etc.; and children or adults who are involved in transition from one life situation to another as, for instance, during admission to care when hazards of physical and emotional stress and dangers of damage arise.

The management of uncertain situations can be considered in terms of the given definitions and it is particularly relevant to do so in relation to recognizable at-risk factors. It is suggested then, that the framework for analysis, although of general relevance in social work, is of particular relevance to action in the dangerous situation.

RISK-MANAGEMENT

Returning to the commercial insurance scene, Williams and Heins (1971:21) suggest that: 'In a broad sense risk management may be defined as the minimization of the adverse effects of risk at minimum cost through its identification, measurement, and control.' One way of discussing the handling of dangerous situations, then, is to follow the familiar line and begin with risk discovery − what are the hazards and dangers? − what are the possible outcomes? − what are the likely outcomes? etc. Within the risk analysis framework some management issues do emerge separately from the questions of predictive ability and decision-making skills discussed earlier.

(1) Uncertainty Management

A feature of the risk situation is the given factor of uncertainty. This uncertainty will create two groups of problems. In the first place difficulties exist because it is never possible to know precisely what will happen in any course of action. In the case of Mrs K, for instance, the social worker cannot know whether the admission of the old lady to an old people's home will lead to a better outcome than not admitting her. The worker may be faced with the possibility of assuring Mrs K that she will be better in a home and taking the risk that when she arrives there she will be unhappy − and therefore be unwilling to trust the worker in further matters. The alternative of telling Mrs K that there is no way of knowing about the outcome carries the risk that she will refuse to go and be exposed to potentially more hazardous factors in her own home. In practice the worker does neither of these but treads a careful line of explanation and discussion which depends on her own authority and confidence in the situation. In an uncertain situation the uncertainty is shared with the client through the worker's own confidence in her ability to help and through a process which might be called anything from 'rational consideration of the current person-situation configuration' (Hollis 1964) to talking about the choices. The imperative is the need to provide the client with full information so that an informed choice can be made: if not for the course of action of greatest benefit, then for the course of action of least potential loss or damage. In a situation of uncertainty, clarification and information giving are necessary.

A second closely associated set of problems relates to the

subjective response to uncertainty. In the face of lack of information or uncertainty of outcome, clients – and workers – may becomes anxious. Perhaps paradoxically they may also become anxious in the face of apparent certainty: if it appears that nothing will happen to relieve a stressful situation anxiety may build up. Mrs K may be anxious because she does not know what will happen if she is not admitted to care but she may also become anxious if, having decided to apply for care, there seems no prospect of a place. A major part of social work is therefore focused on the management of those subjective responses which both the client and the social worker experience when they feel that the outcomes are uncertain. Social work literature is perhaps principally composed of discussion, suggestions, and descriptions concerning this area of functioning and at this stage it is only necessary to relate this within the risk framework.

(2) Manipulation of Likelihood, or Hazard Management

The risk analysis framework identifies the relationship between dangers, hazards, and strengths which already exist in a situation, and those hazards and strengths which may arise if certain courses of action are followed and which may lead to loss or gain. Options emerge which will offer ways of affecting the hazards which make danger a probability. If hazards can be altered or influenced the nature or likelihood of the danger can be affected.

Prevention is possible if hazards can be changed or avoided. If predictive hazards exist in a situation, measures can be taken to reduce the likelihood of specific hazards occurring. For Mrs K the existence of a fire-guard will reduce the danger of her burning herself if she can be persuaded to use it. Hazards can be *prevented*, *removed*, *minimized*, or *offset* by strengths which exist or which are created. Mrs K's forgetfulness is a hazard to leaving the gas cooker on but this can be removed by the addition of a simple mechanical device to the cooker – or offset by the introduction of a memory pad, or a regular routine.

In so far as it highlights the possibilities for affecting the likelihood of a loss (or gain) outcome the risk-analysis framework offers considerable potential. It will also give the opportunity to identify those uncertainties and hazards which can be tolerated, or borne.

(3) Risk-Bearing

Since uncertainty is a given feature of all situations some kinds of uncertainty are clearly tolerable. Social workers and clients are continually involved in making decisions about which uncertainties can be accepted, and lived and worked with, and which hazards can be borne. Mrs K, for instance, may be prepared to accept the uncertainty of her rather precarious existence and to bear the hazards of her present life because she finds these preferable to the unbearable uncertainty of leaving her own home to face the hazards of a new environment. Assuming that she is able to make a rational choice − a difficult concept in itself − she may be preferring the dangers of falling, fire, or heart attack to the dangers of loss of independence, loss of familiar surroundings, etc.

In the same situation the social worker may choose to bear the hazards of criticism from Mrs K's neighbours or daughter rather than expose herself and Mrs K to the consequences of 'persuading' the old lady to go into a home against her wishes.

In this sense, risk-bearing is less a conscious decision between uncertain alternatives, more a choice dilemma − a decision between undesirable alternatives both of which have negative consequences. Whatever decision Mrs K, or the social worker takes, the course of action followed is likely to include uncertainty and hazards for each and they will bear some risk whatever happens. Risk-taking − following a course of action which has a potential positive outcome while recognizing the existence of a potential negative outcome − is distinct from risk-bearing and will be discussed separately.

(4) Insurance

In the social work situation insurance can be defined in two broad ways. In a general sense insurance (or perhaps more accurately, 'assurance') refers to any actions taken to reduce the likelihood of loss and therefore relates to all the actions of the social worker, or clients, which are directed at avoiding the loss outcome.

In a second sense, more closely related to the financial insurance context, insurance refers to actions or measures taken to ensure that if the feared dangers do occur the effects are offset to some degree: compensation is arranged.

The traditional insurance measures are combination, whereby the possible loss is reduced by increasing the number of units exposed to danger, and the transferring of the risk to some other party. It is helpful to consider the social work case conference technique as an insurance measure. In the sense that case conferences pool existing knowledge and help participants to clarify alternatives they are a feature of risk analysis. In that they may help members to control their anxiety about a situation through sharing the decision making – and therefore facilitate a more objective, less pressured approach – case conferences offer uncertainty-management. There remains at least one other potential outcome of the case conference in that actors involved may combine the responsibility for making a decision. If the decision is followed by a serious negative outcome the blame is less likely to fall on one member. The concept of responsibility is an important feature of risky situations in that the social worker may *feel responsible* and therefore feel guilt if loss or damage occurs, or may be *held to be responsible* in a moral or legal sense and be blamed, with perhaps consequent loss of employment. The case conference offers insurance to the individual who can reduce his exposure to guilt or blame through combination with others.

Similarly a group of residents in residential care may combine in demanding a change in practice in the home and share the potential loss – such as deterioration in staff-resident relationships – between them. They are also able to share the common loss of independence, or of family contact which may become subjectively less hurtful if held in common.

The social work supervision situation can also be seen to have insurance elements in so far as the social worker may seek to transfer the responsibility (the hazard to guilt or blame) to his senior. This is not, of course, the only, or the main purpose of supervision but is certainly a feature. Similarly Mrs K's daughter may try to transfer the decision about her mother's future to the social worker: if she succeeds and the feared damage occurs she can then console herself with the thought that she 'did everything possible'.

LIABILITY RISK

In social work two main liabilities exist which relate to the felt or imposed duties of the worker towards his clients.

(1) Moral and Assumed Liability

This makes itself felt in the demands which are made informally on the social worker, as for instance in the limits set by the local community, or by the mass-media response to certain actions or policies. It is also felt in the limits which the social worker carries in his own attitudes, beliefs, and values.

(2) Legal Liability

This will be dealt with in detail in Chapter 4. Some legal duties of social workers are very specifically laid down: this is particularly true of child protection legislation. Other duties are less specific in that they relate to vague criteria of application: whether, for instance a telephone should be provided for an old lady. Other duties are even less clear in so far as they have never been adequately defined: the question, for example, of whether there is a duty to 'protect' residents in old people's homes from specific hazards.

The implication of the existence of liabilities in social work is that there is a strong responsibility element within the risk situation. In some contexts this will be hazardous; at other times responsibility will be a strength.

RISK-TAKING

Risk-taking has been comprehensively defined and risk-taking behaviour has been widely described and discussed. Bem (1971) suggests that taking a risk can be viewed as a selection of one alternative or course of action from among many in which the consequences of that choice could leave the individual in a worse position than if he had selected otherwise or not selected at all. Risk-taking involves a conscious awareness of the relative likelihood of outcome, and the putting at stake of something (in the sense of exposure to potential negative outcome) in the expectation that a possible positive outcome will occur.

It was suggested earlier that risk is a value neutral term but risk-taking behaviour may be seen as exciting or even desirable in certain social contexts. The evidence about behaviour in risky, and dangerous situations is vast and important but cannot be dealt with comprehensively here. One area of the debate which is worthy of mention is taken from the social psychology field and may have relevance for the case conference. It is now well-documented that individual choices on risky problems change following group discussion – frequently, but not invariably towards a more dangerous course of action. This phenomenon is described as risky-shift.*

Although the data on risky-shift is very complex and often contradictory – and it may be that the tests used do not measure attitudes to risk-taking at all (Blascovich and Ginsberg 1978) – some interesting questions are raised about the assumptions made about social work case conferences, and supervision discussion.

Interesting questions are also raised by research findings of bystander response in emergency, or dangerous situations. Latane and Darley (1970:125) recognized certain features of behaviour in what they described as emergencies. They suggest that an emergency has four features: it involves the threat of harm, or actual harm; it is an unusual and rare event; emergencies differ widely in terms of cause and action required;

---

* See *Journal of Personality and Social Psychology* 20 No. 3, December 1971: Special Issue on the Risky-Shift.

and emergencies are unforeseen. In a series of experimental situations, some of which were moderately serious and some of which involved life and death potential they found that bystanders were less likely to intervene if other bystanders were present. This may be, they suggest, because an audience of others inhibits what may be seen as a foolish action; it may be that others serve as guides to behaviour and if others are inactive this provides a model; these two factors together may lead the observer – seeing inaction – to believe that the situation is not serious; and finally they hypothesize that the 'presence of other people dilutes the responsibility felt by any single bystander'. This final point is potentially very important for the case conference situation. If dilution of responsibility does inhibit action (and the reasons to think so are largely speculative) it is essential that decisions are always recorded and action, and actors specified. At this point a further definition can be added:

emergency: a situation in which danger is imminent.

Social workers often take risks in putting themselves in danger in the hope of gain for clients but they also allocate risks to clients who may then take, and bear risks. An understanding of risk-taking behaviour is therefore essential to good practice.

RISK AND ADMISSION TO CARE

In the light of the discussion that has gone before, two questions can now be asked about the relationship between risk concepts and admission to care. In the first place it is important to discuss the relevance of the definitions of risk, danger, hazard, loss/gain, and strengths to the admission process: is admission a hazardous process? – are the likely hazards and dangers of sufficient gravity and probability to justify describing the admission process as dangerous? – and if so is it more dangerous for some people than for others? The second important question is whether the risk analysis framework is a helpful action tool in admitting a client to care. These questions can be explored through a brief illustration.

The N Family

Mr and Mrs N, both aged 23, have been living with Mr N's parents in a three-bedroomed council house since Mr N left the army four months ago. They have two children, aged 2 years and 6 months and Mr N's sister (aged 16) also lives in the house. Tension in the family has built up and on two occasions in the last week Mr and Mrs N and the children have been to the Housing Department refusing to return home but, after being classified as intentially homeless, have eventually returned home. On a third occasion they were adamant and the Housing Department finally agreed to place them in a hostel at the far side of the city. They have no friends or family in that area and Mr N is unemployed.

There are clearly hazards in the existing situation which this family bring to the emergency and to these are added two more sets of factors − those that occur during the admission process, and those related to the new situation in which they will find themselves after admission. Examples of each of these are given in *Table 2(1)*.

TABLE 2(1)

	Predictive Hazards	*Situational Hazards*	*Strengths*	*Dangers*
Existing	Unemployed Youth of Mr and Mrs N	Distress Young children Breakdown of relation- ship with parents	Family together Housing Dept. agree to help	Night with- out shelter Marital stress Loss of sleep Illness, or other damage to children
Admission	Existing distress Moving away from friends	Young children Hurried move/lack of prep- aration	Family together	No food for children Children anxious/ distressed Loss of

TABLE 2(1)—cont.

	Predictive Hazards	Situational Hazards	Strengths	Dangers
	and family Breakdown of relation- ship with parents	Moving to a new en- vironment Difficulty of getting food for children		family and friends Loss of self- esteem
Future	Unemploy- ment Youth No perma- nent home	Away from familiar area Loss of contact with family and friends Difficulty of finding work Children unsettled/ distressed Unfamiliar area	Shelter Family together Access to social work help Free from rows with parents	Marital stress/ separation Mr N will not find work Delay in re- housing Financial loss Loss of self-esteem

The actual process of moving from one place to the next is likely to be more hazardous for the children who will probably be cold, hungry, and unhappy. Mr and Mrs N will probably also experience these deprivations but are less vulnerable to the physical dangers than the young children. A common hazard of admission is that if it occurs hurriedly there may not be proper preparation – in the sense of building up compensatory strengths and reducing potential hazards. The time factor is only one reason why preparation may be neglected. Other reasons are associated with the ability to understand the possible outcomes that may occur during the process.

These outcomes can be identified in the individual risk-analysis framework but can also be discussed in more general terms. In subsequent chapters the risks, hazards, and dangers of the admission process are outlined in relation to recommendations for using the potential strengths in various situations, not just to avoid loss, but also to increase the likelihood of gain.

RISK ANALYSIS AND MANAGEMENT: FINAL
REFLECTIONS

It would be hard to dispute that risk features prominently in British social work. Some attempt has been made here to clarify the component parts of the risk concept in terms of the way it is used in current thinking. Danger and emergency are a major part of the social work job and a clear understanding of these concepts is also essential. It is particularly important to place them within an action framework, or − put less pretentiously − social workers must know what to do to help clients in danger and in uncertainty.

   The risk-analysis framework has emerged from a very small number of basic definitions and does offer a structure for thinking. It owes something to several sources, particularly the problem-orientated record approach which offers, in the medical setting, a way to organize the patient's record logically and efficiently and is said to help the doctor to define and follow clinical problems one by one and then systematically to relate and resolve them (Weed 1969). The framework also owes something to the current search in social work for a unifying theme to link a vast range of component parts. The use of social systems theory to provide this link has received perhaps the greatest attention (see, for example, Pincus and Minahan 1973; Specht and Vickery 1977; Goldstein 1973). This offers a theoretical approach to describing all social work situations and then deriving action possibilities. The risk-analysis framework offers unifying possibilities in that it structures many ways of describing situations and can be used in the individual as well as the general context. Most importantly it provides not just a base for prescribing action but a continuous means of balancing and counter-balancing potentialities within an action focus. The bridge from theory to practice rests on the worker's ability to anticipate possible outcomes and their likelihood, value, and imminence. It links the problem-solving focus to the process view of social work through the interaction between anticipation and action and includes a recognition of the inevitability of uncertainty.

In emphasizing the importance of danger the framework does not ignore the possibility of gain: therapeutic optimism is as much a feature of social work as anxiety about danger. A full analysis will include a consideration of both the potential losses and potential gains which may arise from hazards and strengths. The primary concentration in dangerous situations will, however, be on the potential loss outcome.

3   Admission: Process and
Purpose   *Paul Brearley*

It is not difficult to find descriptions of admission to institutional situations which highlight the negative aspects of the
experience. There can be few social workers who are not
familiar with the feelings of guilt, frustration, and even despair
which can be aroused at having to remove a child, or old person
to care. However good the institution to which they are going it
is unlikely that they will be able to regard it as the ideal, or even
the most attractive answer to the problems of the moment. At
best, admission to care may be seen as the least unattractive
alternative for the person in crisis.

The negative views are evident throughout the range of
institutional provision:

'. . . the admission by parents that they need the help of an
outside agency leads to a loss of status and feelings of
inadequacy, guilt, anger, powerlessness and shame. For both
parents and children, reception into care involves the break-
ing of existing ties and the feelings of loss and grief that
accompany this . . .' (Claydon 1976).

'. . . For the psychiatric patient and the prisoner the worst
part of the procedure may be not knowing what will happen
next, allied to the indignity of being "processed"' (Jones
1972a).

'Admission to any form of residential care . . . implies that
the person has broken down, or broken out, or failed in some
way in his former life' (Berry 1972a).

The ideas of separation, loss, and the anxiety of fear of the
unknown frequently recur in writings about the individual

experience of leaving the community and entry into protected living. The assumption that admission to care is a consequence of some form of failure or breakdown is also predominant. This is clearly reinforced by the suggestions that residential care is a last resort. It may be conceptually attractive to argue that residential homes are in some sense a part of the 'wider community' (Clough 1978) but it is hard to believe that an old lady entering a home and selling her house and furniture will not feel that she is irretrievably leaving behind very important supports. A further group of negatives that are often referred to are those which are experienced at the point of admission. The newcomer is described as being stripped − often physically − of all those things that made up his or her previous self. This may be a substitution of institutional uniform for previous clothing or it may be the divesting of important social roles and resocialization into institutional norms and expectations.

Separation, loss, and exposure to the stress of moving from one environment to another, and to new and potentially stressful experiences can all be seen as hazardous for the person who is in transition. These factors can be explored fully and the hazards carefully examined in terms of the ways that are available to mitigate, prevent, or remove the hazards and thereby reduce the likelihood of loss, damage, or diminution but it is important also to be aware of the potential gains which exist for the newcomer to institutional care:

'. . . the admission procedure could have a potential for introducing the individual to his new environment in a constructive way' (Bradshaw, Emerson, and Haxby 1972).

'Whilst unclear in his own mind whether or not he was mentally ill, an uncertainty I shared, he was clear that he wanted a period of *rest and asylum*, in a psychiatric clinic if necessary, but definitely not under compulsion' (Monach 1978).

In these brief quotations it is clear that institutional care and the admission process are seen to have positive benefits. Foremost among these must be the sanctuary which such care offers: the possibility of rest and relief from intolerable stress is of major importance. It is some years since Jehu wrote that 'it is important to distinguish between "preventing admission to care" and "preventing deprivation"' (Jehu 1962), but the distinction is still as important. To enter institutional care may be hazardous but not to do so may be even more hazardous. The person in transition who comes from a situation of great stress to a new, unknown, potentially safe but also potentially damaging environment is likely to be ambivalent. As one old lady wrote:

> 'I came into this home very suddenly as a result of my sister's death and was totally unprepared. My early impressions were somewhat mixed. I had been living for over 30 years with my only sister, nine years my junior, and found the crowd of folk little to my liking. The noise, exaggerated by my hearing aid, was deafening, especially at meal times, and my sole refuge for peace and quiet was bed' (Anon 1978).

This discussion has so far focused on admission to institutional living but the concept of admission to care relates also to broader issues. It is not easy, however, to define the boundaries of the concept. Many children who are admitted to care live not in residential homes but with foster parents, and although subject to a Care Order, many remain with their own parents. Is it possible, then, to describe children who live for a few days, or weeks, with friends or relatives while their mother is in hospital as being 'admitted to care'? A related difficulty lies in the question of how far Children's Homes can be defined as institutions in the sense that they share common characteristics with prisons, or long-stay psychiatric hospitals. Does the process of admission to a small family-group home for children have features in common with the process of admission to an Old People's Home for fifty or sixty people?

Other complications can be seen to arise from the compulsory nature of some admissions. Is the care provided for a frail and dependent old lady in any way comparable with the confinement of a convicted criminal in prison? Similarly can compulsory admission for treatment to a psychiatric hospital in an emergency be compared to the admission of a mentally handicapped child to a home after a long period of preparation, so that his family can take a short holiday?

Admission to care is not a single concept, or process. It is a term which is used to cover widely differing events and which can include an immensely varied range of experiences. The definition of the term is not easy: the concept of 'care' may include several components, such as 'protection', 'support', 'treatment' or 'containment'. The admission may be to the family group in a foster-home, or to a hospital ward, or even, arguably to a day-centre or day hospital. It is therefore tempting to look for an all-embracing definition. Admission to care might, perhaps, be defined as movement from living in a family or community environment to a protected and/or restricted environment.

Such a definition does not, however, cover the whole field satisfactorily. A care order made on a child, for instance, permits the child to be returned home to his family and in this sense the entry to the status 'in care' does not involve environmental change. It is important to be aware of the distinction between two elements of the possible definition.

(1) Admission to care may involve change in status but not of location. The child who is the subject of a Care Order may continue to live with his family and is involved in a *transition of status*.

(2) In the majority of cases admission to care involves moving to a new environment where care can be offered in the form of treatment, support, protection, or containment. In this sense there is both a change in status and a *transition of environment*.

This book is concerned with the second of these elements: with those clients who are involved in moving from one environment to another. It is particularly emphasized that admission is essentially an individual experience and it is the meaning of that experience to the person in transition which must be of primary concern to the social worker. It has been extensively argued that admission to care is a process of change. In this book it is accepted that this process of change can be recognized and discussed in general terms in the sense that certain types or groups of events are common to all admissions. Nevertheless the framework within which the process occurs is of profound significance and although the main elements of the process itself are common the decisions and approaches made within and in association with the process may vary considerably from one setting to another.

ADMISSION AS A PROCESS

A number of writers have attempted to describe the admission process in common terms: to identify the component parts of the process which can be seen to be common to all admissions. Before considering some of these attempts a number of qualifying factors must be considered. In the sense that admission involves change through time it is a process which can have a beginning, a middle, and an end and these parts of the process may be described in detailed terms. However the point at which the process begins, the approach to the process, and what is seen as the end are clearly influenced by factors such as the urgency of need, the part played by the client in making the decision (how rational, or responsible the client may be), the part played by the social worker in making the decision, the values on which action is based, and the knowledge which underlies the action. To take a basic example the patient admitted under Section 29 of the 1959 Mental Health Act may go through a process of admission but the decision may be made primarily by the social worker, the preparation may be mainly carried out in the car on the way to hospital, and the settling in period may consist of the social worker exchanging a few hurried words with a busy nurse. In contrast, the decision to remove a child from his home may be the result of months of cumulative work and may finally be made by a case conference, not by the worker involved. Preparation may have taken place with the family over an extended period and the social worker will expect to continue working with the child in care. In both cases the process has similar components but these may be extended, or contracted by circumstances: the emphasis on approaches and styles within the process, and on different parts of the process will vary. To be admitted or to admit to an Old People's Home is not the same as being admitted or admitting to a Children's Home or psychiatric hospital although similar stages of assessment, decision making, and action are involved.

One attempt (Billis 1973) to break down the admission process has brought together two important perspectives on the use of residential care. Billis discusses social need within a framework of organizational pressures and is concerned with analysis of problems presented by workers in a Social Services Department with an emphasis on providing solutions to problems. He outlines the process of admission in terms of the key decisions to be made during the process. He distinguishes the decision − of 'undoubted gravity' − which the client makes from those decisions made within the department and identifies eight decisions at the heart of the placement system. The first question is whether residential care is needed or not − a decision which may be regarded as a preliminary evaluation of the client's needs. This is followed by a group of decisions which classify the case: whether it is an emergency, what its relative priority in the area might be; and what its priority throughout the department is. A further set of decisions are then required about the relationship between the need and the resource: whether the client is suitable for the suggested vacancy; and whether the suggested home is suitable for the client. Finally the issue has to be resolved: what action is to be taken?

One perspective on the process, then, sees it in terms of key decisions to be made: the investigation of client need and the matching of that need with the available resources. As has been suggested earlier, however, it is probably as important to know who makes the decision, and carries the responsibility, as it is to know what decisions are to be made.

A further perspective is the now widely known view of admission to care presented by Goffman (1961). He argues that every institution has an encompassing, or total nature which is symbolized by the barrier to social interaction with the outside world and to leaving the institution, which is often a part of the physical environment, such as locked doors, or high walls, or separation from centres of population. The central feature of total institutions as described by Goffman lies in the breakdown of barriers between sleeping, working, and playing: everything happens in the same place, with a group of other people; all phases of the day are tightly scheduled, and all the enforced activities are brought together into a single rational plan. Goffman suggests that the new entrant to this environment is exposed to a process whereby his self is systematically mortified: he is stripped of the supports provided by the stable social arrangement of the life he left behind.

Goffman's descriptions of the mortification of self and of the total institution have received considerable attention and many writers have been able to discuss institutions in similar terms. There is some evidence, however, which casts doubts on the general applicability of the hypothesis to admission procedures in all types of total institutions. Bradshaw, Emerson, and Haxby (1972), in a study of admission procedures in two prisons in England, suggest that 'inmate defacement and mortification' are not in fact used consciously in admission procedures to prison. Where a mild form of 'mortifying' approaches were distinguished they were, Bradshaw suggests, 'more probably the unintentional by-products of a prison-system that is clogged by overcrowding and motivated too exclusively by the primary goal of containment'. An equally important finding of this study was that, contrary to Goffman's suggestion that stable social arrangements are removed by admission, many new entrants came from unstable situations. The prisoner role represented their first opportunity to clearly define themselves for some time.

The general applicability of Goffman's conception is doubtful but it does offer a useful way of considering the experience of admission to care of many people. It may be that many old people who enter residential care do so to escape from crisis and instability but they will inevitably lose opportunities and roles which were previously available to them: the patient or resident role may be a poor substitute for the role of householder, neighbour, etc.

The most comprehensive approach to detailing the component parts of the admission process has been that of Professor Kathleen Jones (1972a). She suggests that the admission procedure to any residential institution can be analysed in terms of at least five sets of theoretical constructs:

(i) as a mortification of self;
(ii) as an initiation rite;
(iii) as a necessary administrative process;
(iv) as a life crisis;
(v) as a socialization process.

In the light of these five constructs Professor Jones breaks down the process of admission into twenty-four stages. She argues, through the comparison of three practical situations, that even transitions as unalike as a confused old lady entering a psychiatric hospital, and a divorced stockbroker planning a holiday in Cannes, have common process elements. Pope (1978) has summarized, rather loosely, these elements into four phases which he calls preparation, separation, transition, and incorporation. It is these four phases which seem to be potentially productive for the social worker and the client during admission.

The process of admission to care – whether to an institution, or to a foster-family situation – involves movement through time. It will begin with the perception, identification, and anticipation of a hazard or danger either by the client or some other in his environment and this is followed by *investigation and assessment*. If admission is judged necessary – whether urgently, or at more leisure – the client must be helped with the *decision* and with *preparation*. There will then be a physical transfer from one environment to another and finally a period of *integration and recovery* (although this latter is the optimistic view: for some it will be a period of deterioration and even death). These stages must be seen within various perspectives: of decision making; of economic or administrative pressures; of socialization and initiation; of time and above all in terms of the meaning of the experience to the individual.

THE PROCESS: BEFORE ADMISSION

(1) Admission as a Helping Resource

From one viewpoint, residential care, foster care, or the psychiatric hospital can be regarded as resources for the field social worker. In this respect it is important for the worker to have tools of assessment and allocation available to him. It has been suggested (Webb 1975) that one method of categorizing or structuring thinking about residential care is to use the approach which emphasizes the difference between thinking of an organization as an 'economic' system, and as a 'social' system. From the economic viewpoint admission to care can be seen in terms of the most efficient use of a scarce and expensive resource to meet a large and diverse range of needs. This view raises questions about the administrative processes by which a decision to admit is made but on a broader basis it also raises issues concerning the type of facilities to be provided, where they are to be provided, and for what type of client. The social care view of resources will be concerned less with the generality of need measurement and more with individual need. It emphasizes the importance of initial investigation and assessment of the client's need and a flexible matching of individual need with resources.

The social worker who uses institutional or foster care resources is concerned with both of these perspectives. He will have to be aware of the generality of need in his area − how the resources can be used to the best advantage for all − as well as the need of the individual client. The decision to admit is not simply about one client and his family but about all the other clients who could benefit from the use of the resources which will be consumed. In this context it is clear that informal as well as formal rationing devices operate. The waiting list for Old People's Homes, for instance, is arguably an effective device for avoiding taking action (Brearley 1972).

(2) Admission as a Crisis Experience

Juliet Berry (1972a) has argued that the client entering care comes from a state of crisis and also that the admission is itself a crisis. The concept of crisis has been given a specialized meaning in social work, and has been defined as an upset in steady state. Rapoport (1965) outlines three sets of interrelated factors which may produce crisis: a hazardous event which poses a threat; a threat to instinctual need, symbolically linked to earlier threats that resulted in vulnerability; and an inability to respond with adequate coping mechanisms. The state of crisis has a fixed time period, usually suggested to be from one to six weeks. There are said to be characteristic phases in the crisis period. In the initial phase there is a rise in tension and if habitual problem-solving mechanisms fail the tension will increase. Emergency problem-solving mechanisms are then used but if they too fail a state of major disorganization may result.

The most important element of this approach to understanding crisis is the suggestion that the crisis promotes the development and use of new approaches to coping. In the crisis situation there are opportunities to learn new ways of dealing with problems and thereby strengthen the individual's adaptive capacity in future situations. Rapoport suggests that certain coping patterns in crisis are maladaptive: for example, regression, magical thinking and fantasy, and withdrawal. Other patterns are essentially adaptive and she lists the necessary response patterns for what she calls healthy crisis resolution. First, there should be 'correct cognitive perception' of the situation: there should be a management and awareness of feelings and verbalization encouraging 'tension discharge and mastery'. Finally there should be a development of patterns of using interpersonal and other resources to help with tasks and feelings.

If the admission process is set in motion when a client is in a state of crisis it is likely that he will be particularly vulnerable in the sense that whatever happens will have an unusually significant effect on him — for good or ill. The process of admission may be a crisis in itself but may also be a continuation of an existing crisis. The fact that admission has been judged to be necessary may be an indication that the client has failed to adapt to an earlier crisis and that failure, or the

belief that he has failed, is unlikely to predispose to the successful management of the admission crisis. Admission to care, in
other words, may be a stressful experience made more stressful
by the loss and distress which the client brings from the
situation which led to the need for admission. The implication
of the crisis intervention approach seems to be in the importance of using the crisis to promote new coping and adaptive
mechanisms through helping the client to understand what is
happening, to cope with the feelings aroused, and to recognize
the potential strengths in the people and resources available to
him.

(3) Admission as a Separation Experience

In addition to being seen as an experience of crisis, admission to
care has also frequently been described as a separation
experience. In so far as the client admitted to an institution is
physically removed from his family or friends for a considerable time he is clearly separated. The term is very closely
linked to the experience of loss and both of these elements have
received careful attention.

Separation has been written about in very elaborate terms, as
in the following quotation:

'Birth itself, our first major experience, is a separation, a
thrusting out from a warm, protective all-providing haven
into a cold and lonely world where needs are not met
immediately. No wonder so many young children sleep in
foetal positions, as if to recapture the feeling of this initial
security' (Lennhoff 1967:3).

Other writers have considered separation in more coldly
intellectual terms but the implication that separation is a
potentially distressing and even damaging experience is predominant. Bowlby (see, for example, Bowlby 1965; 1971; 1975)
is perhaps the most extensively quoted writer on the subject of
separation and children and it has been in the field of childhood
and child care that most research has been done.

Bowlby's early work (1951) emphasized the importance for

the child of a continuous relationship with his mother and of the mothering relationship being warm and intimate. In 1965 Ainsworth, writing with Bowlby, suggested that 'maternal deprivation' occurs when a young child lives in an institution or hospital where there is no major substitute mother and where there is not enough opportunity to interact with a mother figure. It may also occur when the child lives with his mother, or a permanent mother-figure, but receives insufficient care and attention. Another set of conditions Ainsworth identifies as leading to maternal deprivation stem from discontinuity in a relationship, but she points out that a child who is separated from his mother may still interact with a substitute mother. Finally she suggests that maternal deprivation is a term that can include 'distorted' relationships in which interactions between mother and child are regarded as having an unhealthy outcome.

In a discussion of more recent findings on separation responses Bowlby (1975) states that if a child is separated unwillingly from a mother-figure with whom he has been able to develop an attachment he will show distress. This distress will take the form of an initial, vigorous protest, followed later by apparent despair of ever recovering the mother, but the child still remains focused on the mother figure. Finally he seems to lose interest in his mother and becomes emotionally detached from her. Bowlby points out that if the period of separation is not too prolonged the attachment will re-emerge when the mother returns to him.

In a review of research findings in this field Rutter (1972) claims that the loss of an attachment figure is a major factor in causing short-term effects but is of only minor importance with respect to longer-term consequences. The evidence, he argues, strongly suggests that long-term consequences are more likely to be due to a lack of some kind or to privation rather than to any loss. Rutter points out the diversity of effects of a variety of factors which are grouped under the general description 'maternal deprivation'. He distinguishes between the disruption of bonding which probably leads to distress, and failure of bonding to develop which may lead to longer-term damage.

It is apparent from much of these writings that it is the existence of close, emotional ties or bonds between the child and an attachment figure which is important to healthy development in the long term. Separation does not necessarily break these bonds and although it may cause distress, linked to the loss-meaning of the separation, the bonds can be maintained or redeveloped. The findings are clearly important to the social worker involved in admitting a child to care and this will be discussed in Chapter 5. The relevance of the findings to adults who are admitted for care or treatment is less clear. It does not seem unlikely that separation from family and friends will cause distress and unhappiness (although it may also be the cause of some feeling of relief or release) but whether this can have longer-term implications is less clear. It will be suggested in Chapter 7 that the psychological response of old people to the decision to enter a home and to admission is, at least in part, a function of the loss-meaning of separation from their previous situation.

Admission to care, as a separation experience and an experience of loss, is likely to be distressing. Whether or not the distress has a lasting effect, the extent to which the person in transition can make positive use of the care or treatment facilities will be affected by how the distress is handled. The social worker therefore has an important role to play in minimizing the distress (reducing the hazards).

Separation is, of course, a two-sided experience and although this discussion has been concerned with the needs of the child or adult who is admitted, it is equally important to safeguard the rights and needs of those who are left behind. The majority of research has concentrated on 'maternal deprivation' but the concept of 'filial deprivation' can also be considered. Early work made little more than passing reference to the needs of the parents in the child care setting. Britton (1955) developed an approach to filial deprivation and recognized that in all cases where parents have failed to keep their child there is a tremendous sense of guilt which can be completely paralysing. She felt that this sense of guilt and the associated feelings of helplessness can be so great that it could lead the parents to reject the child. More recent work (Jenkins and Norman 1972) has found that all parents experience some form of emotional reaction when their child is placed away from them but that these feelings tend to be focused on themselves rather than on the child. They tend to see admission as a reflection on their own performance as parents and their feelings are particularly self-directed in the form of guilt. One important finding made by Jenkins and Norman relates to the parents' response to separation over time: feelings of relief and thankfulness at the removal of the child tend to increase over time but other feelings have been found to decrease. This has implications for the possibilities of maintaining contact between parents and child. The main emphasis in child care literature has been on the maintenance of some link between natural parent and child although some work has stressed the importance of differentiating between psychological and biological parenting and has warned against encouraging contact with a parent who has only biological significance for the child (Goldstein, Freud, and Solnit 1973).

In the child-care situation the welfare of the child will be of primary consideration and the needs of his parents will be of only secondary consideration. This is not, however, a justification for ignoring the needs of the parents. In other social work situations the primary focus will be less easy to identify. In the case of Mrs K (Chapter 2), for instance, the needs of her daughter – herself approaching old age, in poor health, and with a husband to consider – may be held to be as important as the needs of the old lady. Similarly, if a severely depressed middle-aged man is admitted to a psychiatric hospital the needs of his wife and children may, at least in the short term, be of more importance for the social worker.

In one sense the situation left behind by the person who is admitted is of importance because his family are important in their own right and their material, physical, or emotional distress may demand help. In another sense it is important because of the need to keep open the possibility of return. This may involve work with the parents of a child to enable them to maintain contact whilst he is in care, or it may mean protecting the property of an old lady and making sure her rent is paid in case she wishes to return home.

The rights of those left behind extend beyond the right to be helped with feelings. They have a right − sometimes legal, sometimes moral − to be assured that certain aspects of the care or treatment provided are in accordance with their wishes. On the one hand, for example, this may be the right to prescribe the religious upbringing of their child and on another the right to discuss how far the care of an elderly relative is being carried out in accordance with stated and agreed objectives.

(4) Admission as an Experience of Compulsion

There is a fundamental difference between receiving people into care in the sense that they come voluntarily, or without the use of legal authority, and removing people for care, treatment, or containment with the use of formal, legal authority. Between these two ends of the spectrum − the voluntary decision to enter care, and the legally enforced removal − is a large area of uncertainty. Gostin (1975) has argued in relation to formal and informal admissions of adults to psychiatric hospital under the terms of the 1959 Mental Health Act that an informal patient does not in fact enter or stay in hospital of his own free will if his entry is based on the fear that a compulsory admission will ensue if he does not agree to informal admission. Pressure from relatives, neighbours, doctors, and social workers is frequently considerable, and although many admissions are made without the use of statutory authority it seems likely that many of these are the result of less formal but still real compulsion.

The relevance for the present discussion lies particularly in how far the fact that admission is the result of compulsion can be seen to affect the comparability of the experience to the voluntary admission. One important element may be how far the compulsory admission is experienced as undesirable. It may be a relief to the client to have the decision made for him and far from being distressed at being compelled he may be glad to be free of existing stress. On the other hand some clients may be admitted on the basis of legal powers because they are judged to be unable to make a rational decision.

A further consideration will be how far the client invests the social worker with authority, distinct from his legal, or statutory powers. Power and authority have been widely discussed in social work, although there has been relatively little literature specifically on the subject. Foren and Bailey have argued (1968) that the caseworker's authority derives at least as much from the knowledge and professional skill that he possesses or is believed to possess as from the power conferred on him by society. If the client regards the social worker as a powerful person this will influence the extent to which he can resist the worker's advice or pressure, and will also influence the interpretation of discussions with the worker.

Social workers have a range of legal powers with which to compel people to change their environment to obtain care, treatment, or containment. Many admissions will take place without the exercise of these powers. In 1971, for instance, 84 per cent of the total number of admissions under the 1959 Mental Health Act were informal and 93 per cent of patients resident in psychiatric hospitals had been informally admitted (Gostin 1975). Nevertheless social workers do have less formal authority and between those admissions which are the result of the formal exercise of legal powers and those which are entirely voluntary is a large area in which pressure may be brought to bear from many sources on the individual to enter care. Some of the issues involved in compulsion are looked at in more detail in Chapter 6. For the present purpose it must be pointed out that although the process of admission – involving beginning, middle, and end stages – is similar whether or not compulsion exists, the element of authority is an important determinant of the nature and extent of social work involvement in the process. This will vary from the mental health setting where the great majority of admissions in which social workers are involved will involve statutory authority, through the child care situation in which admissions will be both formal and informal, to the situation of the elderly where relatively few admissions to residential care involving social workers will require the use of legal powers.

(5) Emergency Admission

An emergency has earlier been defined (Chapter 2) as a situation in which danger is imminent. In such a situation action must follow quickly either to offset the pressing hazard or to remove the vulnerable person from the situation in which the hazard exists and therefore avoid the danger.

The emergency is a situation in which the concepts of risk, hazard, and danger are predominant and the analysis of hazards and dangers will assist the worker and client in deciding on a course of action. When the likelihood and gravity of the negative outcome is assessed and its imminence evaluated action options will emerge. There will certainly be true emergency situations when it will be obvious that immediate action is necessary to avoid a disastrous outcome. The old man whose daughter has been admitted to hospital and who cannot care for himself will need help urgently. The homeless family with two small children will need accommodation before the night. In such situations the admission process will be compressed into a very short space of time and there is a likelihood that some elements will be neglected.

It has been suggested (by, for example, Clarke 1971; Jackson 1971) that anxiety during the psychiatric emergency may lead to confusion and apprehension on the part of the social worker and an inability to offer constructive help. Olsen (1977) argues that 'at the moment our understanding of the aetiology of the psychiatric crisis is meagre and our management of the situation remains primitive.' It is particularly important that the stage of investigation and assessment is not neglected as there are certainly occasions in social work when a situation acquires the appearance of urgency through a process of pressure and demand. I have described elsewhere (Brearley 1975), for instance, the process whereby the needs of an old person in difficult circumstances can become an emergency when those around him begin to panic and demand immediate action because of their own anxiety, rather than because of an objective need. Similarly concern has been expressed at the number of psychiatric admissions which are carried out under

Section 29 of the Mental Health Act: in some areas the Department of Health and Social Security reports that such admissions have contributed over 80 per cent of all compulsory admissions (Gordon 1978). When workloads and anxiety levels are high there seems to be a tendency to take hurried action. It is important therefore to distinguish between the true emergency situation in which urgent admission is the only way to avoid damage or loss, and the panic situation in which there is subjective pressure to act in a hurried way but in which objective need is less pressing. The danger of the latter situation is that the admission process will be inadequately carried out and the opportunity to make better use of the caring situation lost or impaired.

The fact that some admissions are carried out in a short space of time does not, once again, alter the nature of the stages in the process but will have an important effect on the social work approach. The time dimension is one more important variable in the process.

THE PROCESS – CARRYING OUT THE ADMISSION

In a discussion of assessment and of moving from investigation to action it is important to be aware of the complexity of value judgements which take place. It is difficult to find concensus in social work on what constitutes basic or primary values or even how the concept 'value' might be defined. One definition describes a value as an enduring belief that one mode of conduct or end-state of existence is personally or socially preferable to an opposite or converse mode of conduct or end-state of existence (Rokeach 1973). A CCETSW Working Party (1976) suggests that a value is used as a socially accepted standard that guides the individual in making choices and that a value can be operative only when the individual knows what he is doing and is aware of alternatives for action and can make a choice between alternatives.

The concept of a 'right way' of admitting people to care involves general values as well as situationally specific values. On a general level, if it is accepted that the basic principle of social work is the recognition of the value and dignity of every human being (BASW 1975) then a concern for the enhancement of human well-being will underlie social work action in helping an individual in distress. One justification, or explanation for social work involvement in the admission process, then, is that it is a potentially stressful and distressing experience. On a more specific level social workers may become involved in admission because they have a legal responsibility; they may be involved with a client on a long-term basis and therefore be a part of his admission process by virtue of that longer-term action; and they may be involved not only because of the past and present distress but because action during the crisis of admission may assist the client to make 'better' use of the caring situation.

Rees (1978) has argued that the provision of 'help' by social workers is dependent, to an extent, on the ability of the client to demonstrate his worthy 'moral character'. He claims that both clients and social workers are concerned with certain values and both groups distinguish between deserving, less deserving, and non-deserving people. It may be, in these terms, that social workers are more likely to offer help in the admission to care, as in other situations, if the client is able to demonstrate the worthiness of his need. As a CCETSW Working Party Report (1976:17) suggests, 'social workers need to be able to examine carefully and critically the values which pervade society and appreciate the manner in which they impinge on their activities.'

The outline of the admission process which follows is based on many value assumptions and rests fundamentally on the belief that the rights and dignity of the individual must be respected however stressful or hurried the situation. The schematic representation is given in only a basic outline form which will be expanded and extended in later chapters.

THE ADMISSION PROCESS

The following stages are involved:

Problem perception
Investigation and analysis
Decision

Preparation
Transfer
Integration
Maintenance and Recovery.

These stages can be elaborated:

(1) A danger is anticipated, or a hazard is perceived or identified.
(2) A comprehensive investigation takes place involving . . .
(3) Consultation between all those concerned – the potential resident, the family and/or significant others; field and residential staff, agency administration, and so on – regarding alternatives.

This facilitates:

(4) The identification of predictive and specific hazards, of potential dangers, and of possible courses of action and the potential hazards and dangers of each course of action.
(5) The formulation of an initial plan of action (admission) which results in . . .
(6) Negotiations in all quarters, and culminates in . . .
(7) Selection of appropriate/available residential unit, or foster-home.

This is followed by:

(8) (Extensive) preparation for admission –
(a) from a perspective outside the unit by the field social worker and the potential resident and family working together; field and residential workers (or foster-parents, or medical staff) working together; and by the field social worker and the agency administration.
(b) from a perspective inside the unit by residential workers (foster parents/medical staff) and field workers working together; residential worker, etc. and potential resident, and family working together; and by the residential worker, etc. and the establishment (management, staff, and existing residents).

So that eventually:

(9) Transfer and reception into care takes place.
(10) Help is provided for the new arrival in understanding the expectations and demands of the new environment.
(11) Support/maintenance, and/or treatment/rehabilitation appropriate to the circumstances is provided within a framework of analysis incorporating an awareness of loss or gain outcomes.
(12) Where possible the aim will be eventual restoration to the community at a more satisfying and satisfactory level of functioning.

The relative importance of aspects of each stage will vary. In the case of the elderly, for instance, it will be shown in Chapter 7 that the making of the decision can be of particular significance. It has been shown that the behaviour of elderly people in institutions, which has been attributed to the effects of institutionalization, begins when the decision is made to apply for care (Tobin and Liebermann 1976). These effects, it is suggested, are attributable to the loss-meaning of separation which begins to have an impact when the decision is made. For the child, however, it is not so much the decision, which is probably made by others, but the actual separation from his attachment figures. For others it may be the impact of arrival at an unknown hospital full of strange smells and unfamiliar demands which is of greatest significance.

The Personal Social Services Council has provided useful discussion documents and practice guidelines for admission to care (PSSC 1975). They make a number of points relevant to admission, relating specifically to adults.

(1) They suggest that every local authority and body providing residential care should draw up a clear written admissions procedure.
(2) They recommend an agreed procedure for assessing the needs and wishes of clients and whether residential care is appropriate. If a decision to admit is made the objectives for the client should be prepared and written down and

written information about the nature and extent of care should be provided.

(3) Decision-making procedures should be established on a shared basis to include the head of home, and the Health Authorities and Social Services Departments should be jointly involved in identifying those at risk in the community.

(4) No final decision about permanent stay should be taken until a review has been carried out after three months stay (PSSC 1977).

The PSSC make extensive recommendations about other aspects of admission and residential care. Perhaps the most important element of their approach is the emphasis on clarity of assessment and objectives. Involvement in admission should be thoughtful and purposeful to reduce uncertainty and anxiety.

THE PROCESS – AFTER ADMISSION

An important question for the social worker is 'where does the admission process end?' One perspective on the mental health admission suggests that the patient admitted compulsorily to a psychiatric hospital is going primarily for treatment and at the point of reception he becomes the responsibility of medical and nursing personnel. This is, of course, not true of all psychiatric admissions and with some patients the field worker will already have and will retain a continuing role with the patient and his family. This situation is, however, rather different from that of the child, or old person where the care, treatment, or containment that is provided is likely to be a resource which is managed and financed by the same department which employs the social worker. Even if this is not the case Children's Homes run by voluntary organizations, or Old People's Homes run privately, or voluntarily are more likely to have social care as their primary orientation. Clearly this difference in orientation is an important factor in determining where the process of social work involvement ends.

In the case of the psychiatric hospital the rights and obligations of the social worker may be curtailed by the medical or psychiatric priorities of the case. In the case of the child, however, a continuing planning and involvement obligation exists for the field worker. Lowenstein (1978) has described the importance of providing a thorough, regular psychological and educational assessment for children in homes, and of the maintenance of a close link (with some exceptions) with a child's family and always with social workers as being among the most important requirements of good care. Similarly, others (Sayer *et al.* 1976) have argued for using positive planning for child placement and for the use of preparation for and follow up to moves as a way of reducing the trauma of crisis and the development of happier Children's Homes.

Parallel arguments have been offered in relation to the elderly admitted to care. The Personal Social Services Council, as outlined above, have argued for follow up and review over at least the initial period after admission. It has also been suggested that once the elderly person has arrived at the home it is important that the field worker does not abandon him and his family at once. There will be a settling in period and to leave the elderly person at this time may only serve to emphasize the feeling of rejection by the community and the feeling of having been 'put away' (Brearley 1976a).

An important aspect of retaining contact with a client admitted to care is the need to keep open the way out of care and back into community living. Some involvement in the child-care setting is a statutory duty but other informal involvement will be focused on retaining links with the family and with helping all concerned to work towards the possibility of living a satis-fying and satisfactory life together in the community. In work with the elderly the focus may be less on work with the inter-personal aspects of the way out and more with the practicalities of home and material supports, and in the mental health setting involvement may be with both the practical and the interpersonal.

For the residential worker the process of involvement may begin at the point of reception but will often have begun earlier with at least discussion of the client's needs. It is sometimes desirable for the residential worker to visit the newcomer in his own home and the residential worker should certainly be involved in the decision to admit a particular client to his, or her home. The way in which the newcomer makes his first contact with his new environment can be of great significance. Berry (1972a) suggests that the transition is often made in a state of merciful numbness. Alternatively many people experience a state of heightened perception and can recall some events vividly many years later. The residential worker has a role to play in easing the difficulties which result from the strangeness and unfamiliarity of the new situation.

Each individual coming into care brings with him a need to influence and affect others: he will want to present and preserve a sense of 'self'. He will also bring with him the distress and sense of crisis from the precipitating event and the process of admission. He may experience a conflict between the need to feel secure and protected and the need to remain a separate, independent being. The residential worker or the foster-parent can help the new arrival by helping him to find a way into the group he is joining. This will require an understanding of the rules of everyday living that operate (achieving socialization) and the exploration of possible roles within the group. In the initial settling-in stage the primary need, however, is likely to be for warmth, and protection within a limiting framework of concern in which the newcomer can begin to recover from his distress and explore the choices for action available to him.

One major implication of the importance of the admission and settling-in period is the need for understanding and com-

together for many different purposes and in its loosest sense the term 'team' may relate to a group of workers meeting together for a specified objective, as in the Case Conference situation. In a more precise sense the team will be a group of people who regularly work together and have formed a close working relationship.

The most difficult person to fit into such a concept of the team is the client. It is easy to lose sight of the client and his rights and it is therefore important that a 'key worker' is identified (RCA/BASW 1976) to take responsibility for each client.

Some concepts can be identified as being of particular importance within the need for effective teamwork. In the first place *communication* between residential workers and field workers is essential if the latter are to be able to retain contact with the client and help with both the settling-in and recovery period. Good working relationships are also important if the field worker is to be able to present a full picture of the client on admission. This can also only be done if good records are available. Residential Homes have been found (Utting 1977) to have good administrative records but poor records on personal histories and reviews. The question of how much information should be shared, and which information can or cannot be passed to different professional groups is, of course, arguable but the importance of clear communication is central.

The relationship between professional social workers and foster parents has also been the subject of considerable debate. The issue of how far foster parents can be regarded as colleagues is important to the way the worker approaches admission to care. It has been suggested (Brimblecombe 1976) that partnership is a word which describes the shared purpose more successfully than the term professional relationship.

These issues of team work, communication, confidentiality, etc. will be discussed in more detail in later chapters. Good practice in admission to care depends on the availability of support, understanding, and trust, as well as on knowledge and skill.

SUMMARY

In this chapter it has been argued that admission to care is a process moving from the recognition and assessment of hazards or potential danger through a decision on action, preparation, and transfer, to arrival and settling in. This process of change through time is similar for a range of settings, and types of admission. It has been recognized, however, that the decisions, and approaches made within and in association with the process are affected by various factors and the time-span and emphases within the process will vary.

Admission has been discussed in terms of its perspective as a resource, as an experience of crisis, and experience of separation and loss, and as a potential experience of compulsion or emergency. Each of these factors, as well as factors in the differing nature of the setting, and above all in the individual experience of the process, will have an important effect on the actions within the process.

Any description of 'good practice' in admission to care raises problems in so far as a generalized position demands extensive qualification. It is also recognized that such a description involves a complexity of value assumptions.

In spite of the difficulties of giving generalized prescriptions for practice in admission to care this review of existing literature and presentation of ideas has attempted to set the scene for the more detailed discussion which follows of the management of admission, and of the associated hazards. There is common ground in admission to care in different settings in two senses. In the first place admission is risky and can be dangerous: existing crisis, compounded by separation and loss, compulsion, and environmental change involve recognizable hazards. These hazards can be identified and the possibilities for taking action to avoid, minimize or remove them evaluated. In the second place admission is a process of change through time involving objectively common stages.

On the basis of these two underlying themes subsequent chapters will proceed, after a discussion of the legal aspects of admission, to a detailed consideration of examples of specific client groups, and of good practice with those groups.

4 Legal Aspects of
Admission *Gwyneth Roberts*

Admission into care is a convenient shorthand term for describing a process which can have a profound effect upon an individual in relation both to his physical environment and to his legal status. Usually admission into care involves movement from living in a family or in the community to living in a protected and/or restricted environment (see Chapter 3, p. 42). If the decision to enter into care is taken voluntarily, the legal implications for the individual are relatively minor. If, however, admission into care takes place as a result of the exercise of compulsory measures then the legal consequences for the individual can be profound.

Social workers are often involved in the process of admitting clients into care since their statutory functions give them power to intervene in people's lives in this way. The exercise of compulsion and control over clients has always been an issue of controversy and concern in social work practice. To what extent should a caring profession be involved in using measures to control clients by taking compulsory steps in relation to them? Quite apart, however, from questions of professional practice and ethics which are discussed in this book, the process of admission into care raises more general issues of principle.

A primary assumption upon which we base the conduct of our lives is that as individual citizens, we should be able to exercise a considerable degree of personal freedom. That freedom is made up of a number of different elements, one of which is the right to move about freely and to choose where and how we live. In other words we assume that we will be free from arbitrary powers of intervention and that the curtailment of our civil liberties will occur only after the exercise of proper authority. Such authority must be derived from the law and must be used strictly in accordance with the terms upon which it is granted. By defining the circumstances in which, for example, a person can be admitted into care, the law also excludes, by implication, all the other circumstances where such action is not authorized so that those who act in abuse of, or without, authority will be accountable for their actions.

It follows that a discussion of the nature and implications of admission into care is incomplete without reference to the relevant legal rules. Without such reference a number of basic questions cannot be answered or at best can be given only partial answers. These questions relate for example to the circumstances in which the process of admission into care can take place, the steps by which it can be carried out, and the implications for the individual client and for the agency of being involved in the process. Sometimes a social worker is involved in the process as a representative of his agency since the legislation may place the responsibility and power in the hands of a local social services authority. At other times, the social worker acts upon authority which has been granted to him by a court, and, at yet other times, the legislation places the authority directly upon him.

Some of the main legal provisions will now be examined in relation to each of the client groups which are discussed in this book – that is, children, the mentally disordered, and the elderly.

CHILDREN

In our society, it is generally assumed that children will be brought up and be looked after by their parents. Human beings are particularly vulnerable in early life and human childhood consists of a long period of dependency during which physical, emotional, and psychological needs must be met if the child is to gain maturity and reach adulthood. It is generally agreed that the best environment for ensuring a child's proper development is that which is provided by the care and protection of his parents within the family unit. To this end, the law reinforces the biological tie between parents and children by referring to rights of custody and care and control over the child.

However, as well as being a private responsibility of parents, the care of children has become a matter of general concern to society for a number of reasons. We recognize, for instance, that most families will need to make use of a range of services in the community to support them in fulfilling their parenting functions. But we also recognize that for a variety of reasons there will be some parents who will not be able to perform their protective and caring functions towards their children in a proper manner and that such failure can result in actual harm to children or place them in potential danger. Over the last hundred years or so, the circumstances in which children are perceived to be in need of protection have gradually been extended and a number of statutory provisions have been introduced, often pragmatically in response to the recognition of a particular need, rather than as a result of the systematic and theoretical development of a concept of social responsibility for children. The result is a somewhat complex body of legislative rules. In effect, however, the law attempts to balance the need to intervene in family relationships where a child's interests are in jeopardy against the rights of parents to look after their children, rights which are supported in principle both by social practice and by legal recognition. The balance which has to be achieved between these two objectives is often a fine one and the conflict which at times results is perhaps inevitable.

One of the important functions of local social services in this field is to exercise protection over children by admitting them into care. They must then ensure that proper provision is made for alternative accommodation for them while in care. Since, however, admission into care is now regarded as a potentially risky step for a child, in relation, for example, to his emotional and psychological development, it has been recognized that local authorities should be able to take steps to prevent it from happening. Indeed it has been suggested that the 'objective of modern family policy with regard to children is to give every encouragement to the family to fulfil its role as provider for the child of sustenance and protection during its vulnerable years and as the primary agency through which the child is introduced into and adapted into the wider society' (Eekelaar 1971 : 143). It has been further suggested that 'therapy is better than surgery, prevention than cure, and that measures have been adopted to relieve pressure upon families at risk while enabling children to be brought up by their families' (Freeman 1974: 19). An acknowledgement of the importance of preventing children from being admitted into care is now to be found in the legislation. Under a duty placed upon them by Section 1 of the Children and Young Persons Act, 1963, local authorities must make available such advice, guidance, and assistance as may promote the welfare of children by diminishing the need to receive or keep them in care or bring them before a juvenile court. In addition, the section gives local authorities power to provide assistance in kind or in exceptional circumstances in cash, in order to fulfil these aims. It also enables authorities to call upon other resources in the community to carry out this function since they may make arrangements for the provision of advice, guidance, and assistance by voluntary organizations or by other persons.

This provision clearly puts stress upon the importance of supportive casework with families with the aim of keeping children in the community and, as Home Office Circular 204/1963 puts it, 'Section 1 has been drawn in sufficiently wide terms to give scope for initiative and experiment by local authorities . . .' A wide range of services can be made available under Section 1, the limitation being often decided by the stringencies of financial and other resources.

Most controversy centres on the payment of cash under the section in order to support families and so prevent children from coming into care. Local authorities differ widely in their interpretation of what are 'exceptional circumstances' where money payments could be made, and also in the amounts which they are prepared to pay under Section 1. There is also the problem which arises from the fact that the primary source of financial assistance should be the Supplementary Benefit Commission and not local social service authorities. Circular

204/1963 indicates that this section was not intended for payments where the resources of the Supplementary Benefit Commission could be used although there seems to be evidence that that does, in fact, happen. Section 1 money is intended primarily for use in emergencies and not as regular payments to families.

For this, and for other reasons, there will be circumstances in which it will become necessary or even desirable for a child to be admitted into care. Sometimes admission will be a direct result of failure of attempts to do preventive work under Section 1, or it will arise as a consequence of lack of the necessary resources to achieve this aim. At other times, the admission of the child can result from a crisis which means that there is no opportunity or time for preventive work to be attempted.

In such circumstances, reception into care can take place in accordance with two quite separate procedures and with quite different legal consequences. These are reception into care under Section 1 of the Children Act, 1948 and committal into care under the Children and Young Persons Act, 1969.

Reception into Care

Local social services authorities must receive a child under 17 into its care if it appears that he has neither parent nor guardian or has been or remains abandoned by them, or is lost; or that his parent or guardian are for the time being or permanently prevented by reason of mental or bodily disease or infirmity or other incapacity from providing for his proper accommodation, maintenance, and upbringing; and the intervention of the local authority is necessary in the interests of the welfare of the child.

The majority of children who come into care under this section do so because of the short-term illness of a parent (12,390 during 1975 – 76) or confinement of the mother (1,942), but other children are received in this way because for example a father was unable to cope on the death or desertion of the mother of the family, or the mother of an illegitimate child was unable to make provision for him. The latter two are cases where it might have been hoped, perhaps, that supportive work under Section 1 of the 1963 Act could have prevented a child from having to suffer the trauma of separation from his parent and it should be noted that Section 1 of the Children Act 1948 specifically states that reception into care should only take place if that is necessary in the interests of the welfare of the child.

The basis of admission into care under the Children Act 1948 is that the child should be *received* into care, and there ought, therefore, to be agreement with a parent that this should happen. It has been suggested (Feldman 1978:89) that authorities may put pressure upon parents to allow a child to come into care under Section 1 of this Act as an alternative to initiating compulsory procedures under Section 1 of the Children and Young Persons Act, 1969. In fact, as is further pointed out, such pressure is most improper as the procedure here must be based upon consent. If circumstances warrant compulsory removal into care then the appropriate statutory procedure should be used.

What are the legal consequences of reception into care for parents in relation to their children? Section 1(2) states that it is the duty of a local authority to keep a child in care until he is 18 so long as his welfare requires it. However, according to Section 1(3) a local authority has no authority to keep a child under Section 1 if any parent or guardian desires to take over his care and, where it appears consistent with his welfare, they must endeavour to secure that the care of the child is taken over by a parent or guardian, or by a relative or friend who is if possible of the same religious faith, or who is willing to bring the child up in that faith.

Can a parent, therefore, recover a child from the care of a local authority at any time? Such a reading of the Act would be in keeping with the voluntary principle underlying Section 1 but in fact the legal position is not so straightforward. In the first place, if a child has been in care for more than 6 months, a parent must give 28 days' notice of his intention to remove the child unless the authority have given their consent and waived this requirement. In the second place, the decision in *London Borough of Lewisham* v. *Lewisham Juvenile Court Justices*

[1979] 2 W.L.R. 513, has now established that notification by a parent of his wish to resume care of the child does not automatically terminate the authority's power to keep a child in care. What it means is that they can no longer rely upon *Section 1* as authorizing them to do so. If it is considered that transferring the child to his parent's care is inconsistent with the child's welfare they must take some further step to retain the child in their care such as passing a resolution under Section 2 of the Act to assume parental rights over him. Alternatively, they may apply to make the child a ward of court if, for example, no grounds for passing a resolution exist.

If a child has been in care for less than 6 months so that notice to the authority is not necessary, or the 28 days have lapsed, must the child be returned to the parent on request in accordance again with the apparent spirit of Section 1(3)? It would seem logical that this should be done. In fact, there is again no simple answer. In the Lewisham case, Lord Salmon was of the opinion that the local authority might 'well consider it to be their moral duty to keep the child long enough to have it made a ward of court', although they have no power to pass a parental resolution under Section 2 and Lord Keith of Kinkel felt that there might well be circumstances such as a pending wardship application or a situation of practical impossibility where no court could reasonably order a local authority to return a child. The result of a child being made a ward of court will be that the court will be able to control all questions which relate to the care of the child, the welfare of the child being the first and paramount consideration. It is, however, the case that a parent as well as any other interested party, such as foster parents, may apply to make the child a ward of court.

The assumption of parental rights under Section 2 can be made on the grounds that the child's parents are dead and that he has no parent or guardian; or that a parent has abandoned him; or suffers from some permanent disability which makes him incapable of caring for the child; suffers from a mental disorder rendering him unfit to have care of the child; or is of such habits or mode of life as to be unfit to have care of the child; or has consistently failed without reasonable cause to discharge the obligations of a parent as to be unfit to have care of him; that a parental rights resolution is in force in relation to one parent who is, or is likely to become a member of the same household as the child and the other parent; or that the child has been in the care of an authority or partly in the care of an authority and partly in the care of a voluntary organization for the previous three years.

Once a resolution under Section 2 has been passed the parent may, within 28 days, serve a counter-notice that he objects to the passing of the resolution. The authority must then make an application to a juvenile court within 14 days for an order that the resolution should not lapse. If no application is made within that time the resolution will lapse automatically. If the court makes an order then it will last until the child is 18 unless it is rescinded by a later resolution of the authority as being in the child's benefit. It is also open to a parent to complain to a court at any time that there were no grounds for passing the resolution or that the continuation of the resolution is not in the child's interests.

By the above steps, an initial reception into care can result in quite dire legal consequences for parents in relation to their children. Section 2 is an exception to the usual rules because a parent can lose parental rights over a child without that decision being made initially by a court. It can be argued, of course, that the grounds set out in the section are quite specific and that it would be difficult for a parent who is able and willing to provide a satisfactory home environment for a child to lose the rights to his child in consequence of his reception into care. But the grounds which allow a local authority to acquire parental rights over a child because he has been in care for three years have been the subject of much criticism on the basis that it can lead to poor social work practice. It should be remembered that Section 1 of the Children and Young Persons Act, 1963 (see above) places the same duties upon local authorities to reduce the need to *keep* children in care. Supportive work to reunite families is, therefore, one of the functions of local social services authorities. Children who were initially received into care as a temporary measure may drift into long-term care, a fact which may also result in their losing their parents' care not only physically but also legally.

Committal into Care

Whereas voluntary reception into care arises because there is no parent or guardian or other suitable person to look after the child or because the parent is prevented from doing so, committal into care, with one exception, arises as a direct consequence of an adult's actual or possible treatment of the child. (The exceptional condition arises where care proceedings are based upon a child's alleged offence.) Committal into care can take place whether the parent agrees or not, and will often be against the wishes of the parent, since the action is normally taken in order to protect the child from parental behaviour which is directly harmful to him.

One of the main methods of committal into care is through care proceedings brought under Section 1 of the Children and Young Persons Act, 1969. There are, however, other procedures which can be used for removing a child from its immediate environment. From time to time emergencies occur and there may be no time to bring care proceedings because the child is in very real danger. The way in which action can be taken swiftly is through the removal of a child to a place of safety. A child may also come into care as a consequence of a prosecution by the police because of an alleged offence, since care proceedings based upon the offence condition are hardly ever brought. The magistrates may commit a child who has offended into care if the offence is punishable, in the case of an adult by imprisonment (Section 7(7)).

Removal to a Place of Safety

Place of safety orders provide a relatively simple method of obtaining authority to remove a child from its home in a crisis. Some of the statutory provisions overlap so that they constitute a battery of procedures which can be used according to the particular circumstances.

The main provision for use by social workers is contained in

Section 28(1). This makes it possible for any person to apply to a justice of the peace for a place of safety order in relation to a child under 17. The applicant must have reasonable cause to believe that any of the first six conditions listed in Section 1 of the 1969 Act exist in relation to the child, and must satisfy the justice that there are grounds for the application. Another useful provision is to be found in Section 40 of the Children and Young Persons Act, 1933. In this case, the application is for a warrant which authorizes a police constable to search for a child under 17 and remove him to a place of safety and also to enter any house, building, or other place named in the warrant using force if necessary. This additional power to enter premises is useful when access to a child is difficult and the use of Section 28(1) is, therefore, limited or even useless. The grounds for the application in this case are that there is either reasonable cause to suspect that the child has been or is being assaulted, ill-treated, or neglected in a manner likely to cause him unnecessary suffering or injury to health; or that an offence listed in schedule 1 to the Act has been or is being committed in respect of him. The offences include incest, cruelty, and neglect, and other sexual and violent offences against children.

Applications in these cases can be made directly to an individual justice of the peace although it has been suggested that it is preferable to seek a place of safety order from a juvenile court if one is sitting. 'There will then be an opportunity for three justices who are members of the juvenile court panel to confer together to determine if the conditions for granting the place of safety order are satisfied'. It is the case, with applications for safety orders or warrants, that the only person who must appear before the justice is the applicant. 'Neither the child nor his parent takes part in the proceedings, nor do they have the right to oppose the making of an order' (Hall and Mitchell 1978 : 42). It is suggested that this example of *ex parte* proceedings, that is, in which only one party is present, is an anomaly in the law since a person's rights may be restricted or lost without his knowledge of the application.

Another group of potentially vulnerable children can be

protected by a place of safety order. These are children who are separated from their parents because they are being privately fostered or they have been placed for adoption. An application can be made under Section 7 of the Childrens Act, 1958, or Section 43 of the Adoption Act, 1958, on the grounds generally that either the person who is, or will look after the child is unfit to do so, or the premises are unsuitable or detrimental to the child. In these cases, the application is by way of a complaint to a court unless there is imminent danger to the health of the child in which case a person who is authorized to visit foster children may apply to a single justice for authority to remove a child at once.

In the above cases, a social worker may well be the person who makes the application for a place of safety order. In the instance of an order under Section 28(1) or Section 7, or Section 43, he may also be involved in removing the child or if the application was made under Section 40 of the 1933 Act, he may accompany the police officer who executes the warrant. In all these cases the child will be removed for up to twenty-eight days to a place of safety. This is normally a community home provided or controlled by the local authority, but it can also mean a police station, hospital, surgery, or any other place which is willing to receive the child (Children and Young Persons Act, 1933, Section 107).

There will be circumstances where other agencies in the community use place of safety or other procedures to secure the removal of a child to safety and the local authority may be asked to provide accommodation in those cases as well. For example a police constable can detain a child under 17 if he has reasonable cause to believe the first four conditions in Section 1 of the 1969 Act exist in relation to him and he can then be placed in a place of safety for up to eight days.

A child may also be arrested under Sections 29, 2(5), and 16(3) of the 1969 Act following the committal of an offence and to secure his attendance at care proceedings or at proceedings to vary or discharge a supervision order. In these cases if the child cannot be brought immediately before a court he may be put in a place of safety for seventy-two hours under Sections 29, 2(5), and 16(3).

During the time when the place of safety order and warrant exists, some decision must be reached as to the child's future. Upon the expiration of that period, if no further action has been taken then he must be released to his parents. Hall and Mitchell (1978:43) have suggested that even in those cases where the order lasts for twenty-eight days it should not, in fact, be left to run for more than eight days. This is because neither the child nor his parents can challenge the facts upon which the order is based. 'The child is taken from his home and the parent is losing custody of the child without having an opportunity to be represented, to make a statement, to present evidence, or to refute the allegations of the applicant'. They suggest that unless compelling circumstances dictate otherwise, a local authority should within eight days have had sufficient time to gather the facts necessary to support at least an interim order even if they are not yet prepared for a full hearing in the matter.

Application for an interim care order during the duration of the place of safety order made under Section 28(1) and (4), is, in fact, open not only to the local authority but also the parents who may hope that the alternative to the making of an interim order will result, that is, the early release of the child. It is also the case that a child, who had been detained under Section 28(2) or Section 28(4), or his parents or guardian on his behalf, can apply to a justice for his release and this must happen unless it is felt that he ought to be further detained in his own interests.

Care Proceedings

Under Section 1 of the Children and Young Persons Act, 1969, a local authority can start care proceedings in the juvenile court which may, if the court so decides, result in the making of an order which will grant the authority compulsory powers over a child. Since, as has been pointed out, there is no general concept of social responsibility for children, local social service authorities do not possess a carte blanche to take compulsory measures in the interests of a child. As a result, care proceedings can only be based upon the grounds which are set out in

Section 1. Indeed, an authority is not bound to search out those children who may be in need of protection but if it receives information suggesting that there are grounds for bringing proceedings in relation to a child under 17 who lives or is found in the area then it must then make enquiries into the case, unless satisfied that such enquiries are unnecessary (Section 2(1)). If it then appears that there are grounds for starting care proceedings, a local authority must take this action unless it is satisfied that it would be against the child's interests or the public interest to bring proceedings, or that somebody is about to bring care or criminal proceedings (Section 2(2)). The other bodies which can bring care proceedings are the police and the NSPCC and if the proceedings are based upon the condition which relates to the education of the child (see below) then it is only a local *education* authority (and not the social services department) which can bring the matter before the court.

The applicant in care proceedings has the task of establishing the existence of two sets of conditions. In the first place, one of the 'primary conditions' must be satisfied, and, in the second place, it is necessary to show that the child is in need of care and control which he is unlikely to receive unless an order is made. The seven primary conditions are:

(1) that the child's proper development is being avoidably prevented or neglected or his health is being avoidably neglected or he is being ill-treated;
(2) that it is probable that condition (1) will be satisfied having regard to the fact that the court or another court has found the condition satisfied in the case of any other child who is or was a member of the household to which he belongs;
(3) that it is probable that condition (1) will be satisfied having regard to the fact that a person who has been convicted of an offence mentioned in Schedule 1 of the 1933 Act is or may become a member of the same household as the child;
(4) that he is exposed to moral danger;
(5) that he is beyond the control of his parents;
(6) that he is of compulsory school age and is not receiving

full-time education suitable to his age, ability and aptitude;
(7) that he is guilty of an offence (excluding homicide).

It is for the court to decide whether one or more of the primary
conditions and the 'care and control' condition has been satisfied, and then to consider whether or not to make an order, and
if so which one. The orders available to the court are a care
order (or interim care order); a supervision order, an order
binding over the parents of the child; an hospital order; or a
guardianship order. (The latter two orders relate to the mentally
disordered.) The general duty of a juvenile court in dealing with
a child brought before it is to have regard for his welfare and
it must in a proper case take steps for removing him from
undesirable surroundings and secure that proper provision is
made for his education and training (1933 Act, Section 44).

If the court is not in a position to decide what order to make it
is possible for it to make an interim order (see above) which will
last for a maximum of twenty-eight days. During that period, a
child or his parents on his behalf can apply to a juvenile court
for the order to be discharged. Or he, or his parents, may apply
to the High Court but if that application is unsuccessful then the
local authority may then allow him to live at home only with the
consent of the High Court. When the child is brought before the
juvenile court at the end of the period of the interim order the
court can either make another interim order or they may come
to some other more final decision in relation to him.

If a court decides to make a full care order in care proceedings, then the legal consequences are that the child remains
in the care of the local authority until he reaches the age of 18
(or in exceptional circumstances until he is 19) unless the order
is discharged in the meantime. During the duration of the care
order, the local authority has power to keep him in care not-
withstanding any claim by his parents. The local authority will
be able to determine what kind of alternative care they will
provide for the child, even whether he should or should not go
home to live with his parents. The authority will also acquire a
great many of the other attributes of parenthood so that only
some rights over the child will remain with the parents.

Since care orders can intervene so drastically in the life of a child and its family and with the rights of a parent over his child, the need for legal safeguards is clear. What part can parents play in care proceedings? Their role in the court hearing is, in fact, somewhat ambiguous.

The two parties before the court will be the applicant, and the child as the 'respondent'. Parents can never be parties to the proceedings although they must be given notice of the hearing and may indeed be required to attend during the whole or part of the proceedings. Since, however, they are not parties to the hearing they may take part in the proceedings only to meet any allegations made against them in the course of the hearing. A parent may be required to leave the courtroom while the child is giving evidence or making a statement, provided that the court informs the person who was excluded of the substance of any allegation made against him by the child so that they may then seek to rebut it.

On the other hand, parents must normally be allowed to represent their children before the court, with the exception of those occasions when the child or his parents are legally represented; or in 'beyond care and control' cases; or if the child requests otherwise. Usually, therefore, the views of the parents can be put forward during the presentation of the child's case. This situation presents the converse to the problems outlined above. It assumes that the interests of the parent and child will always coincide. Clearly there will be occasions when this is not the case, for example where the grounds upon which the proceedings have been brought are alleged non-accidental injury to the child. The situation gives rise to additional concern where a child is too young to express himself or may be unable to give an independent statement to the court. Even if the child is being legally represented, the problem arises for the solicitor in deciding from whom he should take his instructions. In an attempt to meet this problem Section 64 of the Childrens Act, 1975 provides that if it appears to a court that there is or may be conflict between the interests of the child and those of his parents, the court may order that the parent is not to be treated as representing the child or as otherwise authorized to act on his behalf. This section will become Section 32A(1) of the 1969 Act if, and when, it is implemented. Section 32B will then allow the court to appoint a guardian *ad litem* to protect the child's interests where the court has found such conflict exists. Even when this section is implemented, however, in all those cases to which the new section will not apply, parents will still not be able to get separate representation. Neither does the section alter the problem that parents will still not be considered as parties to the proceedings. Clearly the rules of the court need to be altered to allow this to happen, as has been recommended by the Justices' Clerks Society in a memorandum to the Home Office (November 1976). Until that happens, there is still the danger that the child's interests are neglected either because the case becomes a contest between the local authority and the parent, or because the parent agrees with the local authority's decision which is not necessarily in the welfare of the child. Or, in the present situation, a parent's rights may be neglected because he is not a party to the proceedings and therefore unable to present his side of the story to the court.

Even when a care order is made there is the possibility of appealing to a court against the making of the order or of applying for its discharge. Appeals can be made to the Crown Court or to the High Court and an application for discharge of an order can be made to the juvenile court at any time by the child or his parent. If this is refused then no further application can be made to the court until the lapse of three months except with the consent of the court. Following the Maria Colwell case, there is now fresh provision in those cases where an application for the discharge of a care order is not opposed. In such cases the court must order, either before or during the proceedings, that no parent or guardian is to be treated as representing the child or as acting on his behalf unless the court is satisfied that such a step is not necessary for safeguarding the interests of the child. At the same time a court must appoint a guardian *ad litem* for the child unless it is satisfied that to do so is unnecessary to safeguard his interests. By this means, an attempt is made to consider the welfare of the child apart from that of either the local social services authority or the child's parents.

The triangular nature of proceedings which affect children when compulsory measures to protect them are taken are clearly illustrated by care proceedings. The problems which arise in relation to the mentally disordered are rather different but equally difficult.

THE MENTALLY DISORDERED

Although admission into care of the mentally disordered presents the same questions of general principle, the justification for intervening in the lives of adults must be based upon different criteria to those which apply where the protection and care of children is at issue. There is a school of thought which regards any intervention with the liberty of adults as wrong, mainly on the grounds that the only proper justification for taking such action is that the individual concerned has breached the criminal law and, on those grounds, might be liable to imprisonment. The detention of people against their will for any other reason is regarded as a dangerous development. In this country, we have a social and legislative policy which attempts to strike a balance between the freedom of the individual and the need to protect him in those circumstances where he is regarded as vulnerable or dangerous because of his mental state. Whether the balance which is now being struck is in the best interests of the individual or of society is the subject of much current concern and debate.

The first problem which must arise in this field is to define the term 'mentally disordered'. According to Section 4 of the Mental Health Act, 1959, it covers those with mental illness, arrested or incomplete development of mind, psychopathic disorder, and any other disorder or disability of the mind. The terms 'psychopathic disorder', 'subnormality', and 'severe subnormality' are further defined in this section but there is no attempt at defining 'mental illness' and the recent Review Document on the Mental Health Act (Cmnd. 7320) speaks of the 'difficulties of producing a definition that would stand the test of time'. There seems little likelihood at present of a change in the current law in this respect. One critic (Bean 1979:101) feels that the problem of general definitions is that they can become 'catch-all' terms. Alcoholics, drug addicts, and sexual deviants could, and indeed have, found themselves detained as 'mentally ill'. It has been suggested that although the Review Document states that any new legislation would specifically exclude such categories as alcohol or drug dependency and sexual deviancy in themselves, yet 'Nosological categories of mental illness remain sufficiently wide to permit any over-zealous treatment official to find some associated condition, say reactive depression, or anxiety which justifies detention' (Bean 1979:101).

Although retaining the sub-divisions, the Review Document suggests that the terms 'sub-normality' and 'severe sub-normality' cause offence and distress and it is therefore proposed that they should be replaced by the terms 'mental handicap' and 'severe mental handicap', and the definitions widened to include impairment of social functioning as well as of intelligence. It is also proposed that the definition of subnormality be widened. At present it is defined as 'a state of arrested or incomplete development of mind which includes subnormality of intelligence and is of a nature or degree which requires or is susceptible to medical treatment or other special care or training'. The authors of the Review Document suggest:

'A new definition of "treatment" which would make it clear that it included care, training, the use of habilitative techniques and medical care, nursing and other professional help would be more in line with today's perception of the needs of the mentally handicapped whilst still covering the treatment needs of other groups of the mentally disordered' (DHSS 1978).

Finally, it is proposed that the term 'psychopathic disorder' should be retained despite the comments of certain groups such as MIND which is critical of retaining powers in relation to a form of mental disorder which they say is neither clearly definable nor considered treatable. The proposal in the Review

Document is that the words 'and requires or is susceptible to medical treatment' should be removed from the Act.

Clearly, in whatever ways mental disorder is defined, problems will occur. It is, however, far from being a matter of academic quibbling since the inclusion of an individual within the category may have far-reaching effects upon his life.

The second problem which arises in this field is concerned with the kinds of measures which are considered appropriate for the care of the mentally disordered. The policy which lies behind the Mental Health Act, 1959 is that the treatment of the mentally disordered should, as far as is possible, be based upon informal admission into hospital. Indeed, almost 90 per cent of patients suffering from mental illness or handicap are in hospital voluntarily and 95 per cent of residents at any one time are in that category (DHSS 1978:1). What is the legal status of these patients? Do they for example have the same rights to leave hospital as patients who are undergoing care and treatment because of a physical disease? Informal patients, like patients who are physically ill, can discharge themselves at any time, and have the right to refuse a particular form or course of treatment. There is, however, the possibility of being detained for up to three days while an application for compulsory admission is made, if the doctor in charge of the patient's treatment thinks that that is necessary, and also that the grounds for compulsory admission exist. The recent Review of the Mental Health Act (DHSS 1978:1) suggests that since Section 30 could be applied to any hospital patient who becomes mentally disordered it cannot be said to differentiate informal psychiatric patients from others. This is, however, akin to special pleading. It can hardly be said that the possibility of Section 30 being used in relation to them will be a prominent consideration in the minds of non-psychiatric patients, whereas its very existence may seem to psychiatric patients to contain an implied threat of compulsory measures being taken to detain them if they refuse the treatment offered. Furthermore, current government proposals to amend the Act do not propose amending the substance of Section 30 except insofar that it is proposed to shorten the period during which the patient may be detained under the section to seventy-two hours. On the contrary, it is proposed to extend the scope of the section to give a Registered Mental Nurse a 'holding power' of up to six hours to enable a report to be obtained from either the doctor in charge of the patient's treatment or his nominated deputy. This proposal has been criticized on the grounds that it might have been thought that the 'overall aim would be to reduce powers as much as possible not extend them to new occupational groups' (Bean 1979: 105).

It is proposed however to remove the other legislative distinctions between informal psychiatric patients and non-psychiatric patients, such as the power to withhold their mail (Section 134); the power of the Home Secretary in certain circumstances to remove people from this country who are in hospital receiving treatment for mental illness and who have no right of abode here (Section 90); and the ambiguity in the current law as to whether Section 141 which relates to legal actions undertaken by patients also relates to informal patients.

The proposal in the White Paper that all informal patients should be given a written statement of their rights including the right to refuse any particular form of treatment, is welcome. Where a patient's status is changed it is proposed that the patient should be informed in writing within twenty-four hours of that taking place, and in addition that he should be informed of the conditions and rights which are appropriate to his new status. Where it is proposed to give an informal patient treatment which is either irreversible, not fully established, or which carries disproportionate risks, the doctor would be required to seek the express consent of the patient and obtain a second opinion before undertaking the treatment. These proposals will, it is hoped, help informal patients who

'rightly or wrongly, feel themselves to be under a degree of coercion. Others, while not detained under the Mental Health Act, may, because of their mental state, be unable to assert a wish to leave the hospital or to refuse consent to a particular form of treatment. There have also been occasions when it has not been made clear to patients that they have ceased to be subject to compulsory powers and that as informal patients they are free to leave hospital if they wish' (DHSS 1978:4).

Despite the fact that most psychiatric patients enter hospital as voluntary patients, there are still around 20,000 patients annually who enter hospital under compulsory measures. The alternative form of compulsory care, that is, guardianship, is used relatively seldom, and will not be discussed in this chapter. The more important procedures for compulsory admission into hospital will be discussed below.

Compulsory Admission into Hospital

It is in this area that, in the words of the Review, 'it is particularly important that the law is strictly observed' (DHSS 1978:28). As is pointed out:

'However fully legislation may spell out the criteria for the use of compulsory powers under the Mental Health Act and the safeguards against misuse, it is on the individuals invoking these powers that the burden of responsibility for proper use must largely rest. The responsibility is a heavy one in which the protection of the public and the importance of ensuring that mentally disordered people receive the help they need have to be weighed against the very serious step of deprivation of liberty' (DHSS 1978:28).

But, observing the law is not always easy because 'the compulsory procedures are inevitably complex and frequently have to be carried out in situations which are confused and distressing and where urgent action is imperative' (DHSS 1978:28).

This is a field in which social workers are often involved if and when they are carrying out the functions of a mental welfare officer. Since the inception of genericism some social services authorities appoint all their staff as mental welfare officers and they are then able to carry out any functions placed upon them by the Act. In other authorities, specialist teams still exist and the role may then be confined to those social workers who are concerned with the mentally disordered as a group. There has been considerable concern about the former situation because it has been felt that many social workers lack specialist knowledge in the field. To try to meet the problem, the Review Document proposes that certain guidelines should be established on the basis of agreement with professional and training bodies and local authority associations. These guidelines would then be used in the appointment of specialist mental welfare officers to be known in future as 'approved social workers'.

One of the important functions which is placed upon mental welfare officers by the Act, and which is also given to the nearest relative of the patient, is to apply for the compulsory admission of a mentally disordered person into hospital. The role of the nearest relative in applying for admission of a patient into hospital has been the subject of discussion recently since it is felt that there are certainly emotional as well as practical reasons why they are not best qualified to take this step. Nonetheless the Review Document is in favour of retaining their powers since it felt that some relatives might prefer to feel that they are in control of the situation, and because it is felt that they are in the best position to judge when they are unable to cope any longer with the patient. Consequently, the nearest relative would continue to be able to make an application under Sections 25 or 26. However, the current power of *any* relative to make an application for emergency admission under Section 29 is felt to be too wide and ought to be restricted to the nearest relative.

Mental welfare officers may apply for the admission of a patient to hospital if the nearest relative does not wish to do so or if there is no nearest relative. In addition to the power granted to the mental welfare officer by Section 27(1) of the Act, there is a duty to make an application in certain circumstances. The duty arises in relation to any patient within the local authority's area where the mental welfare officer

'is satisfied that an application ought to be made and he is of the opinion that it is necessary or proper to make the application having regard to the wishes of the patient's relative or to any other relevant circumstances. Nothing in this section, however, is to be construed as restricting the power of a mental welfare officer to make an application under the Act' (Section 54).

Taken together these sections give a mental welfare officer wide discretion to decide whether or not to make an application, although, in the case of an application under Section 26 (see below) the nearest relative may object and no action can then be taken except with the authority of a court.

The duties of the mental welfare officer have also been felt to need definition and clarification. BASW has suggested a number of functions (BASW 1977a) but the government, while accepting the value of this, feels it is best done by guidance. It is therefore proposed to amend legislation only to place a statutory duty on an 'approved social worker' to interview the person concerned before making an application for compulsory admission and to make him responsible for satisfying himself that the care and treatment offered is in the least restrictive conditions practicable in the circumstances. This would be further strengthened by a code of practice on admission procedures to cover all the professions involved in this task (DHSS 1978:31).

An application for compulsory admission into hospital made under some sections of the Act is for a relatively short time. Short-term powers can be used to remove a person to a place of safety, for admission for observation under Section 25, and for observation in an emergency under Section 29. Place of safety warrants which are rarely used are a means of entering private premises even without permission where it is suspected that a person believed to be suffering from mental disorder is being ill-treated, neglected, or not kept under proper control; or he is unable to care for himself and lives alone. Application is made to a justice of the peace by a mental welfare officer who, along with a doctor must accompany the constable when carrying out the warrant. A warrant can also be issued where a patient who is subject to detention under the Act is absent from hospital without leave, and entry to the premises has been or is likely to be refused. Section 136(1) empowers a police constable to remove a person from a public place if he appears to be suffering from mental disorder and to be in immediate need of care and control and if the constable thinks it necessary to remove him in his own interests or for the protection of other people. Detention in these cases is for a maximum of seventy-two hours and, unless some other action has been taken in the meantime, the person must be released.

Admission for observation under Section 25 can be made on two grounds. The patient must be suffering from mental disorder which warrants detention for observation (with or without treatment) and that detention is in the interests of the patient's own health or safety or with a view to the protection of other people. Detention can be for up to 28 days.

It has not been clear whether medical treatment can be imposed without the patient's consent under Section 25 and the Review Document proposes that it should be made clear that Section 25 is in fact a treatment section but that stronger safeguards should be introduced to protect the rights of such patients. They should be able to ask for their case to be reviewed, in which case an interview should be arranged within three days and a decision made within a further seven days. A nearest relative should have the same right to discharge a patient in hospital under Section 25 as he does under Section 26 (see below).

Section 29 provides for the emergency removal of a patient to hospital for observation for up to seventy-two hours. This now provides the most frequently used form of compulsory admission. As the basis for the admission is that there is some emergency in relation to the patient it is allowed on the basis of one medical recommendation rather than the two which are normally required. The White Paper proposes that there should be tighter monitoring of its use and a fuller statement required of the reasons why urgent admission is needed. This is particularly welcome since as Gostin has pointed out there is evidence of the over-use of the section and an apparent tendency 'to regard detention as an evil only in proportion to its duration' (Gostin 1975 : 29 – 31).

An application for long-term admission into care can be made under Section 26 of the Act. At present the basis upon which an admission for treatment can be made is that:

(1) the patient is suffering from mental illness or severe subnormality or psychopathic disorder and is under 21; and

(2) the mental disorder is of a nature or degree which warrants detention in hospital for medical treatment; and

(3) it is necessary, in the interest of the patient's own health and safety or for the protection of others, that he is detained.

It is now suggested that the criteria for admission under Section 26 should be changed so that the section provides that compulsory admission should be in the interests of the health or safety of the patient *or* that there is a need to protect others from harm, and for *psychopaths* and the *mentally handicapped* that there is a likelihood of benefit from treatment.

It is also proposed that the age limit of up to twenty-one for compulsory admission of psychopaths and the mentally handicapped should be removed but that in these cases there should be a requirement to certify that the patient 'is likely to benefit from treatment'.

Detention under Section 26 can at present be for up to a year but is suggested that the periods for detention should be halved to six months in the first instance, followed by another six months and then by a one-year period.

Few of these proposals go much of the way in meeting criticisms which have been made of the nature and effect of the current procedures and none can be seen as at all radical. It is not perhaps surprising that MIND called the Review Document 'A tidying up operation in which patients' rights are again being swept under the carpet'.

Safeguards for Patients

Every application for compulsory admission must be supported by medical recommendations from certain 'approved' doctors. It might therefore seem that the current procedures, involving a number of individuals with separate statutory functions would provide a sufficient system of checks and balances. As Hoggett points out:

> 'although the medical grounds for admission are a matter for the doctors, the mental welfare officer must himself be "satisfied" that an application ought to be made and he must consider all the relevant circumstances. These must include not only the wishes of relatives and the protection of other people and the expert recommendations of the doctors, but also his own professional judgement about what is the best solution to the problem' (Hoggett 1976:12; see also pp. 51 – 5).

What if, however, there is conflict between doctors and social workers as to their respective roles? It has been suggested that 'social workers may have great difficulty in opposing psychiatrists' (Gostin 1975:36). It is suggested that this situation arises in part because the ground upon which social workers can professionally dissent to the need for compulsory admission relates to the patient's social situation, whereas in fact it will be the medical diagnosis and judgement of the circumstances which will prevail. Medical judgements, however, have been shown to lack both reliability and validity (Gostin 1975:35 – 42). Perhaps it is not surprising, therefore, that MIND has called for the criteria for formal admissions to be changed. They propose that admissions should be on the basis of 'dangerousness to self or others or to grave disablement', the former being much more open to empirical verification than the current grounds.

There is also the problem of limited judicial scrutiny and review because of the operation of Section 141 of the Act. The section provides that no legal proceedings can be brought against a person acting or purporting to act in pursuance of the Mental Health Act without obtaining the leave of the High Court. The permission of the court will only be granted if it is satisfied that there are substantial grounds for alleging that the person acted in bad faith and without reasonable care. This section constitutes a considerable procedural barrier for patients who would otherwise wish to exercise their normal rights of redress in the courts. The Review Document does not, however, advocate the repeal of Section 141 but proposes only that changes should be made to simplify and clarify the present position.

In the light of the current situation, there is undoubtedly cause for concern as to whether the right balance is currently being found between individual liberty and the needs of both society and the patient himself.

THE ELDERLY

Most elderly people who enter residential care do so without any legal procedures being taken to secure their admission. Whether they always enter care of their own free will may, however, be doubtful since all kinds of social and legal pressures can be brought to bear upon them to leave their homes. Moreover, there is one procedure by which elderly people can be forced to enter care even against their specific wishes. The provision is to be found in Section 47 of the National Assistance Act, 1948, as amended by the National Assistance Amendment Act, 1951.

The section is an interesting one because its history is tied up with that of the Poor Law and with public health measures since it seems to have found its way into legislation as a method of facilitating slum clearance (Grey 1979: 19), and as a method of dealing with a possible source of disease and infection arising from unsanitary conditions. It is now the community physician (previously the medical officer of health) who initiates action. He must undertake a thorough inquiry and consideration of the person's situation and decide if it is necessary to remove him either in his own interests or to prevent injury to the health of, or serious nuisance to, other persons. He may then certify his findings in writing and must, if possible, obtain the consent of a manager of suitable premises to take the person in.

The local authority, which in this case will be a district council or a London Borough, may then apply to the local magistrates' court or it may authorize the community physician to do so. The person to be removed or the person in charge of him must be given seven clear days' notice of the application.

The grounds for making the application are that it is necessary to secure care and attention for the person concerned because he is:

(1) suffering from grave chronic disease, or being aged, infirm or physically incapacitated, is living in insanitary conditions; and

(2) is unable to devote to himself proper care and attention and is not receiving it from another person.

The court may make an order of up to three months which can thereafter be renewed indefinitely.

In some circumstances it is possible to remove a person without giving him notice. In this case the community physician and another doctor must consider that it is necessary in the interests of the person to remove him without delay. In this case the application can be made either to the local magistrates' court or to a single justice under Section 1(3) of the National Assistance Act, 1951 to have the person removed. In these circumstances, the order can be made *ex parte*, that is without the person being present before the court or even being represented.

It is not known how many orders are made under Section 47 since no national statistics of its use are kept by central government. It is thought, however, that its use varies from authority to authority depending perhaps upon the personal feelings of the community physician for the area. It seems to be an example of a measure which can be used to deprive an individual of his right to live in the community but about which very little is in fact known.

SUMMARY

The issues which are raised by the compulsory admission of clients into care highlight the tension which must inevitably exist between the concept of freedom of the individual, on the one hand, and the concept of welfare and protection on the other. They are questions which lie at the very heart of social work and it is important that social workers should acknowledge them in their day-by-day practice, since they affect the lives of their clients so profoundly.

Part Two

Introduction   *Paul Brearley*

This discussion has so far been concerned with two particular themes. In the first place risk has been identified both as a key concept in social work but more importantly as a major factor in decision making and action. Second, admission has been explored as a process of change through time. In addition, it is clear that social work decisions and actions are increasingly bounded, if not constrained, by legal responsibilities and requirements.

In the second part of the book these themes are developed in relation to specific situations and to their implications for social workers. Each of the following four chapters has been prepared by a different author and it is perhaps inevitable that each has a different emphasis. Nevertheless each clearly shows that the social worker must take great care in helping the client and his family make the decision to enter care and, if the worker has to make that decision for them, then it must be made in the light of as much information and with as much preparation as possible. The risks of admission are considerable and it should be quite clear that admission is potentially less damaging than other possible courses of action. Similarly, each chapter shows the importance of managing the actual transition from one environment to another with care and with the minimum of disruption.

Peter Marris (1974) has offered a useful debate about common threads in the experience and perception of loss and change, emphasizing particularly the impulse to defend the 'predictability of life' as a fundamental and universal principal of human psychology. Certainly responses to change, in the form of grief and adjustments, can be seen to have common elements in all ages and, perhaps, in all major life changes. There are many similarities between the needs of the elderly, of children, or of the mentally ill (or, indeed, of the mentally handicapped, the disabled, or the homeless, etc.) at the time of admission. All face a difficult decision, and all are involved in important life changes. It is, however, important to recognize the differences. Old people are not 'like children', just as the needs and capacities of children are different from those of adults and each of the chapters on Children, The Elderly, and Mental Health presents background information distinguishing each group. What must also be remembered, of course, is that each individual within those groups is different: it may be possible to talk generally about the needs of children – but each child requires separate consideration.

The final chapter considers the relationship between policy and practice, with special reference to the example of the elderly, through an exploration of different forms of service. That the elderly were selected as the example was entirely fortuitous – the points made by Glenys Jones apply equally to provisions for other groups. The chapter acts as one more reminder that, although the needs of the client are of primary importance those needs exist within, and are partially defined by, the services that are available to meet need. Sadly, the decision that a person, whether young or old, 'needs to be admitted to residential care' may actually mean that there is nothing better at the time, rather than that it is an ideal solution – although it may mean that residential care is a useful and acceptable form of help for that person at that time.

A particularly important point which is frequently referred to in subsequent pages is the relationship between field and residential social work (and social workers). Admission to care may be an end to one part of a person's life but it also a beginning: residential workers and field workers must work together during and after admission to ensure that it is a positive and helpful beginning.

5 Admission and Children
Penny Gutridge

INTRODUCTION

In a population of 55 million the UK has approximately 3,380,000 children under five and nearly 15 million under eighteen; there are some 120,000 children in care in the UK as a whole and, of the 100,000 children in care in England and Wales at the present time, about 40,000 are in residential care (see Manning 1979).

It would appear then that there are a large number of children experiencing the admission process at first hand: having their home situation investigated and assessed following some kind of crisis; being prepared for separation from their parent(s) and for placement with strangers; being physically moved from one place to another and subsequently helped to recover from, to digest, and integrate this experience so that it begins to make some sense in the broader context of their lives.

For some, the process of admission will have been paced and measured with breathing space available for building new relationships, exchanging information, exploring feelings, and maintaining a degree of autonomy and understanding about the process, its purpose and possible outcome. For others admission will have been compressed due to prevailing pressures, with no advance warning and little time for preparation, resulting perhaps in distorted perception of events for both the child and his parents. In either case, the danger of permanent damage to the child cannot be overlooked.

For the majority of children their stay will be brief (Packman 1973), yet it seems that there are more children in care than ever before and, with fewer young children involved, that those coming into care are getting older and staying longer (Parker 1978). This has implications for both community based and residential social workers in terms of the tasks to be undertaken with and for children.

Authorities in child care social work have examined the subject of admission to care already, as a specific area of concern (Jehu 1963; Lennhoff 1967; Claydon 1976) and as part of a larger child care canvas (Timms 1962; Kastell 1962; Pugh 1968; Stevenson 1978a; Bettelheim 1950). There is discussion in the literature about what this experience can mean for children and their parents (Littner 1956; Trasler 1968; Stevenson 1963a; Moss 1966) and for the receiving agency's field and residential social workers (Hudson 1975) and its administrators (Billis 1973; Payne 1976). References mentioned here and drawn upon subsequently in this chapter are just some examples of a persisting professional concern. However no comprehensive study yet exists, and this is surprising given the potential significance of admitting a child to residential care for all concerned (Stevenson 1963a).

Admitting childen to care seems to be a hazardous business for everyone, not least for social workers in whom it can arouse a myriad of feeling associated with their own childhood and parenting experiences perhaps combined with feelings of guilt and failure, powerlessness, anger, and self castigation (Moore 1976). These feelings are by no means exclusive to the admission of children but perhaps the more acute in this instance because of the child client's size, vulnerability, and dependency upon adults for protection and security. Given that the subject is so emotionally charged and so prone to evoke discomfort if scrutinized too deeply, perhaps it is not so surprising that no major work has yet appeared primarily concerned with all aspects of the admission to care of children, and that so much research remains to be done – for example, into:

(1) the factors impinging upon planning, organization, delivery, and upon quality of services to children and their families at the time of admission;
(2) possible discrepancies between ideal and actual social work

practice, perhaps based upon existing practice guides (Jehu 1963; Lennhoff 1967; Claydon 1976) − that is whether discrepancies occur, if so why, and how the situation might be improved;

(3) social work activities with parents and extended families after separation from their child(ren), what might be anticipated and upon what social work intervention might most usefully focus.

Kay explored the impact of removal of a child upon family cohesion for example (Kay 1970) and found a high proportion of accelerated breakdown in parental relationships, separation, and subsequent deterioration in the fathers' circumstances − but I can find no evidence of further study despite the apparent connection with such serious social consequences and likely additional burden upon social and other services.

(4) retrospective consumer opinion − even the National Children's Bureau's young people's working group, when recalling reception into care, confined themselves to reasons for admission, omitting any references to the actual event (Young People's Working Group NCB 1977).

One thing that has emerged very clearly from the available perspectives and which is of paramount importance is the need to focus primarily on the child − legally, professionally, and morally. The tasks facing a child coming into residential care have to do with mastering feelings first, about separation from parents, second, about going to live with strangers, third, about the possibility of separation happening again and so fourth, about the risks involved in getting too close to anyone new (Littner 1956). The social work task is to help children to tackle their own tasks and to help the other people in their lives − those relinquishing them and those receiving them − to play their parts to the best of their ability for the child's sake.

A particularly important issue, then, is the nature and extent of the social worker's role with the child. There is evidence that social workers have been reluctant to offer direct casework help to children (Winnicott 1964, 1977; Holman 1966) and a variety of possible reasons for this have been offered. Space does not permit a full consideration of this issue here but detailed readings are available elsewhere – Timms and Itzin (1961), Vann (1971), Moore (1976), and Thomas (1977). The basic principles and techniques of communicating with children, how to recognize opportunities and make use of them, how to use oneself, other objects and artefacts, and appreciate the limits of what can be achieved are to be found, for example, in the works of Fraiberg (1957), Britton (1955), Timms (1971), Winnicott (1977), Berry (1971), Moore (1976), Rich (1968), Barnes (1978), Stevenson (1963b), and ABAFA (1977). Some inspiring examples of actual practice appear in texts by Turner (1968), Holgate (1972), Younghusband (1965), and Stevenson (1978a). Given energy and imagination such accounts of social work in action might suggest all kinds of improvements for admission practice.

Against the background of this primary need to recognize the child as the focal point of need I shall now consider first, the needs of children, admission and its potential dangers, and second, the admission process.

THE NEEDS OF CHILDREN, ADMISSION, AND THE DANGER OF PERMANENT DAMAGE

The necessity for admission to residential care places a child at risk in that he is exposed to the danger of permanent damage in consequence of hazards likely to be encountered during the process itself, and afterwards. These hazards compound those already negotiated as part of his life so far. We know too that artificial group living can be hazardous and that the child remains at risk in the institution. The way the admission process is handled through its various stages, and subsequent field and residential work practice, can either increase or decrease the likelihood of damage; thus informed and sensitive hazard management by all those receiving the child into care will be vital.

One of the first points Jehu (1963) makes concerns investigating the advisability of admission in the case of a particular child, and Pringle (1975) gives us clear indications of what to expect if a child has to come into care. Brief separation will be at best unsettling, at worst a deeply disturbing and damaging experience, whilst the consequences of long periods in residence may be devastating to social, emotional, and intellectual functioning. However, it is not that physical separation from families, or living in institutions, are necessarily destructive in and of themselves. Drawing upon earlier works (Dinnage and Pringle 1967a, 1967b; Pringle 1971) Pringle points to three major advances in the last quarter century in understanding the implications of substitute care for children. First, that adequate physical care is not sufficient to ensure satisfying emotional, social, and intellectual growth. Second, that prolonged institutional life in a children's home can have a damaging effect upon all round development. Third, that many children could remain in their own homes if effective and sufficient supportive services were available in the community. Roughly half the total number of children coming into care do so because of mother's confinement or short-term illness and a further 10 per cent because of the mental or physical illness, desertion, or death of one or other parent. No two children react the same way to separation (DHSS 1976b; Bowlby 1975) but susceptibility to damage and resilience in the face of actual or apparent rejection − survival in other words − appear to depend largely upon the quality of relationships available to the child in care. Pringle continues that since most children coming into care are likely to be already disadvantaged socially, backward intellectually or educationally, and disturbed emotionally − and so even more vulnerable to permanent damage − it will not be sufficient for residential life to provide simply good physical care; if that is all there is then any positive gain is likely to be limited. Only if children's institutions become therapeutic communities, she says, aiming to remedy and rehabilitate the hurt, confused, and damaged child, can they claim to provide a viable form of substitute care. Minimizing predictive hazards then is a major part of the residential social work task as is the evolving of caring systems (Hunter and Ainsworth 1973), and the establishment of creative living environments for children in line with the thinking of practitioners and writers like Bettelheim (1950), Beedell (1970), Trieschman, Whittaker, and Brendtro (1969), and so many others. Otherwise, the likelihood seems to be from Pringle's study of long-term separations, that children are prone to suffer language and intellectual retardation through, for example, lack of stimulation and personal attention and with consequent effects upon educational performance. They may be less able to express themselves or to function adequately socially compared to their peers. They may also manifest heightened behaviour difficulties in the Home and at school, characterized by frequent irritability, a marked tendency to be miserable, tearful, destructive with their own and other people's belongings, aggressive, and unable to concentrate for any length of time on either work or play — the latter being just as vital for future development and adjustment (Ingram 1961; Winnicott 1971).

Perhaps most worrying of all, however, is the prediction about damage to the growth of self awareness, sense of identity, and personal worth. It has been said that 'partiality' is crucial to a child — that is that some one person in his life will go, not just to reasonable, but to unreasonable lengths on his behalf — and that to be deprived of this seems to be so damaging that it may not be possible ever to make up for it artificially (Newson 1971). Add to this uncertainties about why he came into care, where various important people in his life are now, and what the future is likely to be and one begins to see how pointless it must seem, and impossible it may be, for a child in care to generate life energy and harness available assets. In the words of Brill and Thomas (1964) 'no real group life is possible to a child who has abandoned the hope of intimacy with a beloved adult person.' A child needs to feel that he matters to someone and is valued for his own sake; if lasting and unconditional care and loyalty from an adult are never experienced then the child may fail to develop loving qualities himself and may find it increasingly difficult to trust adults or reciprocate affection (Pringle 1975). Put succinctly, in order to survive, kids, like the rest of us, need at the very least one other person to love them unconditionally — but their need is more urgent and if unmet has graver consequences.

These findings underline the need for social workers to exercise great care in assessing the quality of a child's relationship with each parent, and where this is valuable and valued, to minimize the dangers by ensuring support to keep that relationship secure. Alternatively, where this relationship is missing, impoverished, or lost, they need to seek substitutes such as residential social workers, foster or adoptive parents – even be prepared to offer it themselves if the quality of relationship evolved through shared crises indicates the wisdom of this. The importance of not allowing children's lives to drift in care and of adopting a much more positive, even aggressive approach to substitute home and parent finding is well documented (Rowe and Lambert 1973; Bacon and Rowe 1978; Shaw and Lebens 1978).

Since unmet need is so risky it would seem to be important for social workers to be clear about what children's basic needs really are. Only then can they anticipate the extent of a child's loss and make effective attempts to control and minimize it and to identify strengths in his situation upon which to build both immediately and in the long term. Talking to a child will be one way of discovering his priorities and what is important to him. Apart from this, we know from Pringle (1975) that children need love and security; special opportunities for new, envigorating, and enriching experiences; praise and recognition as unique valued individuals capable of satisfaction in personal achievement; opportunities to exercise responsibility and make positive contributions to their surroundings and their fellows. In Maslow's 'hierarchy of need' (Maslow 1962) physical security – a roof, food, and clothing etc. – take precedence and emotional and spiritual needs follow behind. Brill and Thomas (1964) point out that the question of need can be approached from many angles but that in their opinion emotional needs take priority as directive forces in the child's growth to maturity – though with adequate regard to other factors. Could it be then that for children the 'hierarchy of need' should be redesigned? Drawing upon ideal family life, Brill and Thomas identify six prime necessities:

(1) a close and continuous relationship with one person who

will provide bodily care in such a way as to attach the child's love and admiration, stimulate trust and assurance, and the desire to become like that adult;
(2) a father figure;
(3) a small community life in a reasonably stable group;
(4) opportunity for diversity in activities, possessions, occupations, and leisure;
(5) access to a larger community, or neighbourhood, in whose life he can participate;
(6) an affectionate, stimulating, controlling, and understanding environment in which his urge to become progressively independent will be tolerated and encouraged.

Berry feels the needs of children are deceptively simple. Physically they need a small share of a dwelling and neighbourhood, some food and clothes, a safe warm place to sleep, a few toys, and an occasional wash. Emotionally and socially they need some love from adults they regard as their own, who want and accept them for themselves and treat them consistently so that they develop a sense of security and continuity. Intellectually they need stimulation, opportunities for play, achievement, and discovering themselves in relation to the world at large. It is likely she says that these interconnected needs, though apparently simple enough to satisfy ordinarily, become virtually impossible for parents who were themselves chronically unsatisfied in childhood and whose current needs are so pressing that they find it difficult to recognize or meet the demands of their children. As Berry so accurately observes, unhappy children with unmet needs are far more difficult to look after whether by parents or anyone else (Trasler 1960; Berry 1972).

There is a fair measure of consensus then as regards a child's basic needs and the consequences if these go unmet, or if their fulfilment is disrupted by an upset in his steady state – be the change brief or prolonged. The work of Heinicke and Westheimer (1965), Bowlby (1975), and Rutter (1972) provide examples of the sources of knowledge and prescription, both explicit and implicit, that have been invaluable to social work over the years.

Dinnage and Pringle (1967b) found that large families with low incomes, those where there is only one parent, or where there is some form of handicap are at greater risk of disintegration and that once such a family splits up reintegration is likely to present problems. Thus a child extricated from especially hazardous circumstances via an admittedly hazardous process (admission) to another situation of more than average hazard (residential care) would seem to be particularly endangered.

Jenkins, however, points to shifts in thinking in recent years and to an increasing store of evidence that separation from parents need not have disastrous effects. In the case of brief separation, for example, Rutter's work suggests that events immediately preceding separation may be more damaging than separation itself, and that as regards severely traumatic and prolonged deprivation this can be compensated for by good experiences in later childhood (see Jenkins 1978). The foster care guide to practice (DHSS 1976b) outlines a child's needs and goes on to discuss the broader implications of these and how the individual needs of a child in care can be successfully matched in substitute homes by 'good enough parenting' and skilled foster care practice, and recent studies by Triseliotis (1979) provide additional evidence. Since hope is an essential ingredient for all concerned (Smaldino 1975) we can therefore consider the stages of the admission process in a more positive frame of mind, alert to the hazards, yet reassured that all need not be lost for a child when his relatively steady state is upset and he has to come into care; that management of hazards, risk taking, and putting something consciously at stake in the hope of gain and on the basis of what is tolerable for everyone, can build up a measure of insurance for a child against the danger of permanent damage, associated stress, and unhappiness.

THE STAGES IN THE ADMISSION PROCESS, CRISIS
INTERVENTION, AND HAZARD MANAGEMENT

Important events such as separation, and associated suffering, are part of all our lives and indeed children must separate from their parents at some time (Jenkins 1978; Mason 1968) but for a child and for his parents, each in their own way, admission may well overload their normal coping mechanisms. To acknowledge that a child is experiencing stress is painful for adults (DHSS 1976b) – parent or professional – and we are inclined to defend ourselves by, for instance, denial or flight (Stevenson 1963b). Stevenson has also said however that a social worker must suffer anew each time a child comes into care, suffer with the child and with his parents; that familiarity must never breed contempt or indifference and that we should never seal ourselves off from the experience by denying its impact or meaning for those involved. Each time, she says, we must remain sensitive both to the feelings of others and ourselves, and seek to observe freshly in each case what it means to the individuals concerned (Stevenson 1963a).

Disciplined and skilled use of empathy will be of particular relevance then in emergency situations where facts must be explored quickly and the true nature and extent of the risks identified, when an understanding of the precipitating stresses must be achieved swiftly and accurately, and some assessment made of the adaptive capacities of all the key individuals – why they haven't been able to cope and what strengths they can still bring to the situation. In a state of crisis where habitual problem-solving patterns prove inadequate and where a solution is sought outside the usual problem-solving repertoire, crisis theory can be especially helpful. We know that felt crisis may trigger off old unresolved conflicts between and within people. We know too, however, that it mobilizes energy for coping and mastery, energy that can be harnessed to advantage in negotiating hazards – for example, during the admission process. Crisis theory assumes that the natural progressive tendencies in human development prevail over regressive ones and that a social worker using all the usual casework principles and techniques but accepting a rather more authoritative, temporary leadership role on the basis of his knowledge, expertise and competence can be of value by:

(1) anticipating a client's needs and the tasks he must face;

(2) encouraging the individual(s) concerned to focus on the present and, to a lesser extent, on selected past events and future orientation;

(3) attempting, by means of reality-based reassurance, to lower tension, redefine the problem in manageable terms, help the individual towards mastery of some segment of the experience, and hence re-establish a measure of self confidence and self esteem.

Crisis intervention aims to conserve and restore functioning and even to promote growth through adversity. The prime objective for the social worker will be to reduce anxiety and tension, instil hope of mastery, and by engaging all members of the nuclear family in the helping process, by conveying commitment and optimism, to develop as soon as possible a tentative working hypothesis from which they can all proceed (Roberts and Nee 1970).

The stages of admission are not mutually exclusive of course, they overlap with an obvious midpoint at the time of actual reception, of physically moving from family home to residential unit. In terms of the social work task and hazard management the stages of (i) investigation and assessment, (ii) preparation, (iii) transition, and (iv) integration and recovery blend in a network of interlaced strands – a dynamic that as it progresses will affect the individuals concerned differently in every case and on every separate occasion.

For the purposes of this chapter I have worked on the assumption that admission will be to residential care, and will continue to do so, though in reality, a social worker will – as Jehu (1963) puts it – assess the advisability and legality of admission to care, weighing the desirability of various alternatives against what may happen if the child comes into residence; he will then work towards getting the best bargain he can for the child from the alternatives available. As soon as possible he will work towards a preliminary long-term plan for the child's care away from home. This will mean helping the parents to appreciate the implications of admission, for the child and for themselves, so that they can engage in joint planning with a view to finding and agreeing upon a suitable placement and beginning preparations to ensure continuity of care for the child. Not all parents will be willing or able to cooperate, but ideally social workers will be working towards partnership with a child's parents. Key factors in the planning operation will be first, the worker's knowledge of residential facilities and professional personnel and second, the respective, and hopefully complementary, needs of the child and his family. The need to establish and nurture warm, trusting relationships with parent(s) and child alike cannot be overstated if help is to be pertinent and effective throughout the admission process – and later, as plans for the child's future are reviewed and reformulated, and collaboration with parents to combat damage and maximize possible gain continues.

How matters proceed from the point of referral will depend a great deal on worker style, but the following considerations seem particularly important. No apology is made for approximating to an ideal; the existence of a variety of constraints is readily acknowledged, the contention being, however, that approximation to an ideal is an essential prerequisite of good social work practice.

Although stages of investigation, assessment, and preparation are inextricably bound together, at the outset the worker is inevitably on a fact-finding mission. Formal social history and note taking however will undoubtedly detract from the human interaction so vital to effective practice, and in addition such formalities may grate upon individuals who find themselves both under the stress of actual or impending crisis, and also faced with a powerful official who they may fear will judge them unworthy, ineffectual parents and remove their child summarily. There is growing evidence that clients dread first encounters with social work personnel and are prey to debilitating fantasies as to possible outcomes Reith (1975) – and not without cause it seems (Smith 1975; Rees 1976). Helping people to appreciate the realities of the situation, and at the same time conveying reassurance and hope, begins with first encounters and involves the worker's whole approach. The first imperative is to make it clear who he is, where he is from, and how he can be reached before he parts from parents and child for the first time, otherwise confusion and anxiety may be heightened instead of eased. Next it will be important to know, regardless of the source of the referral, what the parents' views and wishes are. This makes it possible to explore their reasoning and discuss with them whether admission is advisable or even necessary. It allows for discussion about the needs and current predicaments of key individuals, especially the child(ren), and about possible alternatives to residential care. Parents may not have conceived of the range of possibilities the worker will be able to suggest and it may be that with support and encouragement they can evolve a solution for themselves either within the family or neighbourhood network, or with help from community and social services resources. Another crucial issue is whether the child's home is in jeopardy either because of eviction, or likely marital breakdown, or because a parent's life, or mental or physical health, is in the balance, for this will influence how the worker proceeds and the emphases he adopts in subsequent hazard management.

If the child has been admitted to care before, then with continuity of care for the child in mind, and in the interests of a comprehensive social history the worker will want to know:

(1) how long ago?
(2) why and under what circumstances?
(3) by whom, from whom?
(4) from where, to where and for how long?
(5) the extent of parental involvement throughout?
(6) the extent of parental contact during the stay (visits, phone calls, letters, post and birthday cards etc.)?
(7) the circumstances of the child's return home?
(8) what the child thought about it all?
(9) what the child expects now as a result of his previous experiences?
(10) does he expect to return to the same place with the same outcome and is this realistic?

This may be the stage at which a child beyond infancy can be drawn into the deliberations. Whatever his age, even in adolescence, he may remain peripheral to admission planning, with adults talking across and around him unless the worker makes a conscious effort to include him in some way appropriate to his age, level of understanding, and verbal ability. Parents may need help and encouragement to understand the importance of this and to find ways of helping the child to participate. There is evidence however that even very young children can benefit from direct help as a number of writers testify (Timms 1962; ABAFA 1976) and the Robertson film *Kate* so ably illustrates (Robertson 1968).

As part of the data collection it will be essential – again in the interests of continuity of care for children – to know whether the child has siblings elsewhere, if so where they are and whether the family is involved with any other social work or allied agencies – in their current, or any other locality – and whether they are on an 'at risk' register. Inter-agency communication may be crucial to ensuring appropriate planning and avoiding crossed wires which may add to the danger of damage to the child.

By now the social worker will begin to form an assessment of family strengths and weaknesses, including the strength of nuclear and extended family bonds. He will also have some idea of just how hazardous the process is going to be for the child, the parents, himself, and his residential work colleagues – even agency administrators who may become locked in an intra-agency battle over placement alternatives, hinged upon a financial expediency versus professional criteria debate (Billis 1973). Yet another hazardous obstacle for the worker to negotiate!

Everything about the way the worker operates will affect hazard management and this will be reflected in the way he uses time. How soon the child must go and whether the admission process will be compressed, or can be paced over a period of time, may have great significance for mobilizing the child's capacity for mastery. The anxieties and expectations of parents in the grip of felt crisis may lead to the child being swept along on a tidal wave. To avoid his being dashed upon the rocks the worker may have to try and resist prevailing pressures and manoeuvre for time. This will enable him to slow the pace and give the child space for adjustment and preparation; to give himself opportunities to establish and consolidate necessary relationships; to prepare the child for the move and what to expect and help parents to do their part in this; to secure the fullest possible social history, because children's parents can disappear or be lost by default; to prepare those on the receiving end and if possible arrange a prior meeting between child, parents, and residential worker(s); to see teachers, nursery, day care, or playschool staff; to arrange for the health visitor or doctor to call at the child's home where parents have a measure of control over medical formalities; and to give the child time to say goodbye to friends and let them know his new address.

Ideally these things should be carefully planned and timed to suit each particular child's needs. In the case of paced admissions the worker will be able to discuss options with the child and order priorities with him in collaboration with parents. Once a residential unit is decided upon, introductions can begin — though this raises the debate about when residential workers should first be involved in decisions about placement, whether the child should be seen before any decision is made about admission, or reliance placed upon the field worker's submissions. There is no blueprint for introductions but it may be particularly helpful if the residential worker can be introduced to the family on their own territory first. From then on the extent and emphasis of the respective roles of field and residential social worker as regards the child may suggest itself, and who is to be the key worker may emerge as part of the course of events that follow (see RCA/BASW 1976).

An appreciation of the quality and history of the child's relationship with each parent now begins to form; how they feel about the child going; the extent of their guilt or relief, anger and hostility, or shame and sense of failure. The worker will have clarified whether or not both are biological parents to the child, the psychological significance of each parent to the child and vice versa.

It now becomes even more essential to ensure that information is exchanged; that the process is two way and that parents and child feel able to ask questions, clarify and reclarify what will happen, when and how. It may not be possible for anxious parents, or those who are conceptually or emotionally limited to think beyond reception. This means that information about visiting, about the child's life style in residence, how plans for him will be reviewed, decisions made and implemented, and what's expected of, and hoped for from them, may have to be reinforced after the child has moved – perhaps repeatedly.

The exchange of information will include:

(1) what the child needs to know;
(2) what the parents (and extended family?) need to know;
(3) what the school (or nursery, or day care centre, or play-school), the GP, and any other inside or outside agency personnel need to know;
(4) what the residential social work staff and existing children in residence need to know;
(5) what the field social worker *still* needs to know from (1), (2), (3), and (4).

Hopefully the parents will engage with the worker in planning, decision making, and preparing the child for transition to their fullest capacity. The worker's skills will be extended already in helping them to mobilize what strengths they can for the child and one another, and to hold onto whatever positives or hope exists in the situation. He will want to know about the family's routine and about anything specific in the child's lifestyle which could be maintained whilst he is in care; for example, nap or quiet times, bedtime stories, favourite TV programmes, and interests, clubs, and associations. Worker and parents will want to explore together whether parents themselves can ensure continuity in any particular way and so be assured of continued involvement with the child and a tangible degree of autonomy. For example, father and son going fishing or to football matches together, parents and child shopping and buying clothes etc. together, regular visiting to a purpose, attending – and perhaps calling – reviews. Much of this will depend upon agency policies and practice making it possible to follow the basic principles of placement noted by

Hazel (1978) — (i) normalization, or the right to lead a normal life in the community, (ii) localization, the right to develop local roots, (iii) voluntariness, or no coercion except where the child is endangered, (iv) participation, the right to be committed and to share decisions, i.e. implying both parent and child.

Investigation, assessment, and preparation now begin to merge with transition. There are things parents can do to ease transition and at the same time acknowledge and master their own feelings. These include their involvement in the choice of placement, overall planning, and preparation; their commitment to preparatory arrangements and to ensuring that the child is assured of their welcome at the residential unit; preparing his clothing and belongings — ensuring that new purchases do not outnumber familiar items; arranging 'freedom from infection' formalities themselves; clarifying financial obligations — assuming that parents will contribute provides an opportunity for tangible evidence of their care and concern. Parents may wish to accompany the child, stay for tea, put him to bed, and field and residential work colleagues working in harmony will want to ensure that the needs of the institution and rites of passage on reception do not impinge upon the differential needs of particular parents and children (Bradshaw, Emerson, and Haxby 1972; Berry 1972a) and that flexibility in routines and staff attitudes makes it possible to accommodate them — with due regard of course to the needs of the host children.

What is being said to the child, out of earshot of the worker, about prevailing circumstances will now become clearer, whether parents are able to accept and put into practice good intentions, or feel obliged to deal in half truths or deception — either to protect the child, divert, pacify, or punish him. However carefully prepared, Littner (1956) suggests children invariably hope against hope that the need for separation will be averted. As reception nears the worker may be able to tune in to any misapprehensions. It will be vital to ascertain whether or not the child will be afraid to leave home, either because he's been in trouble and fears that loss of parental affection will accompany separation, or because parental ill health, marital strife, dire financial straits, or threat of eviction arouse fears that his parents may be lost to him altogether. Such fears, real or imagined, will need attention.

Detailed records are a must in child care social work and may prove invaluable for someone tracing origins in later years; to fail in this respect is to add to the danger of identity damage.

Often overlooked in preparation are children's precious belongings, especially pets, and experience teaches that a child's attachment to an object or an animal may be an essential link to the past. Not to recognize this and act accordingly can mean total loss of hope for a child. Imaginary friends, for example, may have enormous significance for a child's mental health and the worker who fails to acknowledge this important extra individual and duplicate admission arrangements does so at the child's peril.

An essential ingredient to all four stages in the admission process is some form of child study – not just age, sex, race, colour, religion, national and social origin, but also the stage of development he's reached, some assessment of his assets and deficits, any special characteristics such as any handicap, especially if it is not visible (for example, petit mal), whether he wears spectacles or a hearing aid, has dietary, speech, or toilet problems, his fears and phobias, likes and dislikes, whether his race or religion imply special needs (for example, as regards hair care, food specifications or feast days to be observed lest he feel disloyal to home and parents), health and medical history, such as genetic difficulties in the family, any hereditary illness or special medication, and whether he is in the middle of a series of inoculations or dental treatment. Such a study should also include comments regarding school preoccupations or problems, and whether any treats were imminent and missed on admission (for example, family weddings or anniversaries, or school outings).

The child may be feeling acutely ambivalent towards his parents; perceiving them to be under stress and apparently powerless to rescue him from the axe, he may feel responsible and bad yet angry and resentful, his longing to console tangled up with his need to be consoled and rescued from the inevitable.

He may want to open or widen communication channels with his parents and may be able to use the worker's help to do so.

Ways of helping a child master his own feelings and fulfil his needs for more relaxed and satisfying communication with his parents at this time will depend once again upon the worker's style. Ideas include, for younger children, the use of finger puppets or pipe cleaner dolls, a couple of simple cardboard open-plan dolls' houses, and a toy car (or vehicle similar to that in which the child will travel to the children's home). The suggestion is that these might be used in play to explain pre-ceding events at home and to enact, and re-enact, anticipated events. Toy telephones can be useful for helping little children understand the worker's role as link and resource person, to reassure about and plan continuing parental contact, and give children confidence in future use of the instrument. Paints, coloured crayons, felt pens, and flip charts can help older kids to construct wall charts and posters depicting home, the journey into care, and the residential unit, together with all the important people and things in their life. If a child can be encouraged to work on something like this, perhaps with his parents, he can pin it on the wall at home and use it as a talking point and later it can be reassembled in the children's home, or kept by or for him, as a lasting record, reminder, and tool for reflective discussion. Not all children like to work with paints however and others may prefer leggo or meccano models, plasticine, or papier-mâché as a means of self expression, or to make a scrapbook with picture cut-outs from magazines. Such projects, especially if they involve parents or a teacher as well as the social worker, can facilitate questions and answers and a reliable exchange of information. For some older children and adolescents diaries or autobiographies might be started under the worker's supervision as part of a contract between them and as a means of 'keeping people, places and events alive and relatively unclouded by fantasy' (Winnicott 1964). These too could be held in safekeeping by mutual agreement.

Children want to know how long they are going to be away from home and again truth will be essential, however painful, and time − that precious commodity in social work − must be given to staying with a child's grief and helping him find and consolidate the positives in his life.

Moving from the familiar to the relatively unknown will be stressful (Bettelheim 1950; Lennhoff 1967) however well prepared the child may be. Even when he has visited more than once with perhaps an overnight stay, and initially met residential workers on his own territory, actual reception into care is still peppered with uncertainties for him. How he gets there, who accompanies him, and the way the journey is used to help him master feelings and fears (Stevenson 1963b) will all be significant in terms of how well he can cope with each new threat and challenge. He may need to be reminded about who and what to expect, about names, routines, and any important house rules, about what is likely to happen tonight and in the next few days, and when and how he can contact his parents and friends. If he is going some distance it may be useful to take time out to buy postcards of the new locality with him for immediate posting and giving his new address.

How he is greeted will be of great significance to him and workers should think carefully beforehand about the best time of day to arrive both from his viewpoint and that of other children. Young children in particular may be acutely sensitive to noise, smells, and the sheer size of the place and numbers of people to whom they are expected to relate in rapid succession. It may be wise therefore to consider arranging arrival for a calm, quiet time of the day when other children are either at school or otherwise preoccupied and the key residential worker has time to give unobtrusive, individual attention to the child — to his initial welcome, refreshment, introduction to his room, bed and locker, to ensuring privacy whilst he unpacks and explores. All this assumes close cooperation between field and residential workers, that the child's arrival is expected, carefully planned in advance, and tailored to his special needs. It also assumes that duplicate files have already begun to which each worker will subsequently be contributing.

A number of writers have deplored the depersonalizing and damaging effects of ritualized reception into institutional care (Goffman 1968; Bradshaw, Emerson, and Haxby 1972; Berry

1972a). They cite initiation rites such as form filling, listing possessions, removing and replacing clothing, assigning quarters, and informing about regulations as generally programming the individual out of his individuality and into submission to the institution. At one time children in care were similarly treated – being stripped, deloused, bathed, medically examined, photographed, fed into and spat out of the administrative machine to join a mass of identically uniformed other children and dependent for information upon the subcultural grapevine. The recollection of one man, in conversation with the author in 1975, of his own admission at the age of 5, in 1926, is illustrative. 'I felt as if my identity had been stripped from me with my clothes . . . all they left me was my birthday suit and they could have had that too for all I cared . . . I felt I was nothing, nothing at all . . .'

Whilst routine and limits are undeniably important, rituals such as these at a time of dazed, or perhaps heightened, perception of details and their personal significance have no place in child care social work. A child needs to find his own level in new surroundings with new people, and to go through any necessary formalities, like being cleaned up, in his own good time – though with due regard to protecting the health of other children of course. Belongings should never be thrown out because they're dirty or unhygienic – in a few days, when he's had time to settle in and talk it over he may find it in his heart to give his permission for this. The needs of the institution are also important but they cannot be permitted to crush personal dignity. It may be that someone associated with the child's home should stay with him awhile, perhaps through his first meal or bedtime, ideally a parent or relative but otherwise the social worker with whom he came. It will be important for him to be able to identify with a particular residential worker whom he has met beforehand and who can introduce him to his peers, beginning perhaps with one child although this will depend on the size and composition of the unit. This worker can ease introductions by telling each something about the other in advance, thereby preparing both. Bettelheim refers to 'feeling tone' and the fact that it is not what is said so much as actions and attitudes which colour the newcomer's impressions on first encounter (Bettelheim 1950), whilst Lennhoff cautions against an overpersonal approach – a possible result of identifying too strongly with the child's apparent bewilderment or stress. He says the child who loses his home, even temporarily, is in mourning and has a right to brood, and supportive effort that is not offered with tact and respect for his grief may be experienced by him as intrusion and convince him that nobody really understands (Lennhoff 1967). Thus, there may be two extremes in failure to empathize: (i) not to try; and (ii) to overshoot the mark.

Both Bettelheim and Lennhoff discuss initiation into the peer group as does Berry (1972). They all stress the importance of preparing the group to receive the newcomer and of acknowledging the implications for them of the admission of an additional member in terms of first, the initial concentration of attention on him, second, the subsequent sharing out of attention that will be required, and third, the fact that new arrivals remind existing residents of their own admission and stir old memories and feelings with which they may need help. Bettelheim notes that most newcomers are far more interested in, and concerned about, the other children than adults. They are likely to learn more about the true climate of the unit and how secure and hopeful they can allow themselves to feel, from observing children in interaction with staff and one another than from any other source. He notes that a well-integrated group will probably meet the newcomer with friendly indifference, explaining what they're doing and inviting him to join in, but carrying on much as before, secure enough to take him or leave him. Children of a less well-integrated group may either exclude him, or be openly hostile, or compete avidly for his friendship. Alert residential workers will attempt to anticipate the dangers and offset the hazards here – perhaps, as Bettelheim suggests, enlisting support from the peer group in welcoming the newcomer, for example, by planning together for a special tea and, without making him a central figure, using it as a treat for everyone, and an ice breaker.

Efforts to help a new child settle and integrate are not

confined to the first day however. Recovery from separation, reception, and associated feelings takes time (sometimes forever) and some children take weeks to surface and begin to make any identifiable progress. However, direct work with the child, and indirect work on his behalf will continue inside and outside the residential unit. The residential social worker will be just as concerned with mental health, personality growth, and ego building as with physical care. He too will be concerned with what Beedell (1970) has called integrity provision – that which encourages the development of healthy individuals by adapting sensitively to them, attempting to heal the hurt and damage that's occurred already, and contain any further danger of permanent ill effects.

Trasler (1960) identifies a trinity of pressing needs at this stage – for (i) support, (ii) information, and (iii) an arena for constructive social learning. Meeting the need for support will depend upon the quality of relationship the child has been able to build with his key worker, and whether there is still someone who will go to unreasonable lengths with him in mind but without rivalling his parents or making him feel that he has betrayed them in any way. As regards information, Trasler again reminds us that because children are often dazed or shocked by admission, memories get muddled. Despite prior efforts to prevent 'the tangled web we weave' the worker may be well advised to consider repetition but using a different tool or technique. As Britton (1955) said, much child care social work involves working backwards and it may help to work backwards with the child through play by compiling a scrapbook or constructing together an autobiographical account of his admission in retrospect. This way of imparting, clarifying, and repeating information against a backcloth of loving support fulfils the third element of Trasler's trinity of need by providing the arena, or means, of learning and mastery.

Between them, and according to the roles and responsibilities decided upon, field and residential workers will be offering a comprehensive service of the quality the family will have come to expect since the admission process began. We have a degree of knowledge about filial deprivation and know that parents too may go through stages of protest, despair, denial, and detachment on separation from their children (Jenkins and Norman 1972). Loss of the child himself compounded by loss of autonomy and decision-making powers in respect of him, plus lack of continued interest, support, and encouragement from social workers may lose parents for the child forever. A flexible plan of action to which parents can subscribe provides continuing impetus and a context for regular review. If the child is to be in care for any length of time then some form of review will be required at the end of the first month and certainly within three months. Thereafter reviews can be called as and when necessary but at least every four to six months. Any child able to verbalize should attend his own reviews and key workers should be prepared to go to unreasonable lengths to ensure the presence of at least one parent or relative, or failing this someone from outside the agency who can act as an advocate or ombudsman for the child (Davis 1978). Who defines the need for review and according to what criteria poses an interesting debate but perhaps the child, the parents, and the ombudsman should be encouraged and enabled by social workers to call reviews as they see a need. The 'Who Cares?' and 'Voice of the Child in Care' groups might usefully explore the implications and mechanics of this.

For the child in care, restoration to the community is a certainty sooner or later. What will be at issue when reverse transition and associated crisis is experienced (Godek 1977) is whether he will be a 'restored' individual, i.e. a reasonably happy person, able to function confidently and liking himself well enough to be able to love at least one other person and his own children (Picardie 1970; Pringle 1975).

Debating the concept of 'childhood as destiny' Fraiberg says that adaptive mechanisms in each child's personality are at work very early, acting upon experience in ways that are unique for this personality, and the product in the personality depends ultimately upon the ego and the mode of adaptation and not on the experience itself. Danger to humanity, she argues, lies in diseases of the ego (isolation, detachment, emotional sterility). These happen early due to the absence or destruction of human ties; consequently we have reason to fear 'the hollow man' unattached and unable to give what he has never received and learned from personal experience (Fraiberg 1959).

Social workers – in the community and in residential settings – accept a heavy and joint responsibility when a child is admitted to care. Perhaps good practice can contribute in some small way to preventing these children becoming 'hollow men'?

6   Admission and Mental Health
Frank Hall

Although this chapter is specifically concerned with factors involved in the part the social worker plays in the assessment and admission processes relating to the mentally ill, some explanation should be given of the view indirectly expressed here of more general questions associated with the subject of mental illness *per se*.

The debate about the existence, causes, and nature of mental illness has been going on for a very long time, and a great deal of effort on the part of researchers from a wide range of professional disciplines has been devoted to pursuing their various lines of enquiry. But mental illness stubbornly remains, despite all the attention it has received, largely an enigma with no explanation so far put forward of the fundamental questions it raises being sufficiently strong to oust its competitors. It has, for example, been variously argued that the cause of mental illness is to be found in intrapersonal conflict, interpersonal conflict, faulty learning of behaviour, psychopathogenic families, repressive societies, and cultural moral cowardice. These and other theories and models have contributed a great deal to the understanding of human behaviour at a theoretical level, but have mostly proved disappointing in what they have to offer in practical, and practicable, terms to those confronted with the immediacy of human suffering associated with mental illness. As Pearson has observed 'radical theories do not find their radical practice . . . their moral and political imperatives remain, by and large, things to be read about in books and scholarly essays' (Pearson 1977:203).

The focus of criticism for the more radical theorists is frequently the so-called 'medical model', a model which,

Strongman suggests, 'is so much a part of everyday discourse that it is often forgotten that it represents only one (arbitrary) way of looking at things; it is just a model' (Strongman 1979:46). Nevertheless, the development of services for the mentally ill in this country has mainly been within the Health Service structure and it is within the terms of the medical model that mental illness is most likely to be formally recognized, defined, and treated. In addition, the law relating to mental disorder, including mental illness, with its emphasis on medical rather than legal judgement reinforces the primacy of the medical model. It is for these pragmatic rather than empirical reasons that it is the medical model of mental illness which is used in this chapter.

Features of the medical model which should be borne in mind in the discussion which follows are:

(1) illness is defined in the form of a diagnosis, by a doctor;
(2) the illness itself is believed to be something which *happens* to an individual, for which he and others cannot be blamed and for which the cause is assumed to be natural;
(3) the doctor has the authority to confer the sick role on the person identified as being ill.

Siegler and Osmond (1974:102), following Parsons, identify four important elements in the sick role: a sick person is 'exempted from some or all of his normal social role responsibilities; he cannot help being ill and cannot get well by an act of will; he is expected to want to get well as soon as possible; he is expected to seek appropriate help . . . and to cooperate with that help toward the end of getting well.' As we shall see, in the case of mental illness the sick person can have the decision to seek help taken out of his hands and be legally compelled to receive care and/or treatment. It is this element of compulsion which can be introduced into the mental health situation which is possibly the most difficult for social workers to reconcile to their professional ethic, as it would seem to be contrary to one of the profession's most basic principles − client self-determination. The question of compulsory power and the potential for conflict it creates is discussed at length below, but it is useful to quote here the National Association for Mental Health (MIND) working party report on in-service training for social work with the mentally ill, which recognizes the dilemma with which social workers can be faced: 'The working party felt that all social workers have problems in balancing responsibility to society and clients, with the statutory requirements of the agencies in which they work . . . In work with the mentally ill, social workers have to accept that they have to be caring and concerned with patients' rights, but also have to exercise a degree of direction and control on occasion' (MIND 1976).

With this brief outline of the general viewpoint of mental illness taken here the discussion can now go on to consider the role of the social worker, not in the defining of mental illness, but in assessing the hazards and dangers consequent upon its recognition and ways in which the risks created can be reduced.

ADMISSION: THE SOCIAL WORKER'S ROLE IN
DECISION MAKING

In 1976 a total of 190,358 people were admitted to psychiatric hospitals and other treatment facilities providing for the care of the mentally ill in England and Wales (DHSS 1978). A government white paper published in 1975 (DHSS 1975) suggests that each year some five million cases of diagnosable mental illness are seen by general practitioners and, of these, about 600,000 are referred to the specialist psychiatric services. A graphic demonstration of the significance of these figures is the white paper's suggestion that, on the basis of their figures, one in six of the female population of this country and one in nine of the male population will, at least once in their lives, become psychiatric inpatients. However, these figures cannot be taken as accurately indicating the incidence of mental illness in the population; they reflect only the number of people seeking medical help and the diagnostic practices of the services to which they present themselves. However, for present purposes it is sufficient to accept that, irrespective of the real numbers of mentally ill existing in the community, about 500 people are admitted each day for reasons associated with mental illness.

If we look at the significance of this for social work we can reasonably suppose that as most (88 per cent) of these admissions are informal, they will be effected as an exclusively medical procedure and will neither need nor require the involvement of a social worker. It appears to be equally reasonable to suppose that most of the more than 22,000 formal admissions *will* involve some degree of social work intervention. Unfortunately, we do not know how many informal admissions social workers participate in or how many applications for formal admission are made by relatives. Nor can we assess the influence of social work involvement on the course of events and subsequent outcome; for example how many potentially formal admissions are eventually effected informally (and vice versa) or how many admissions are avoided altogether as a direct result of a social work presence. Such deficiencies in our knowledge must raise questions about the assumptions made above about the numbers of formal and informal admissions involving social workers but, in the discussion which follows, whilst the main emphasis will be on admission and not the legal status of the mentally ill person, a good deal of space is devoted to questions relating to the use of compulsory powers.

The 1959 Mental Health Act lays certain duties, responsibilities, and expectations upon the Mental Welfare Officer (social worker) as well as granting him certain powers. An important requirement made of him is that he does not concentrate solely on the needs of the person thought to be or identified as being ill; he has also to consider the wishes and the welfare of relatives and of society generally. Section 54 of the Mental Health Act reads: 'It shall be the duty of the mental welfare officer to make an application for admission to hospital or a guardianship application in respect of a patient . . . in any case where he is satisfied that such an application ought to be made and is of opinion, having regard to any wishes expressed by relatives of the patient or any other relevant circumstances, that it is necessary or proper for the application to be made by him'. A problem for the social worker in fulfilling this obligation is to determine the relative importance of the possibly differing needs of those involved; does he give priority to the manifest needs of the person designated mentally ill, the needs of the relatives, or the needs of the community? Can the interests of each be served simultaneously and, if not, whose come first? In short, who is the client? Such questions can be the cause of considerable difficulty for a social worker when the nature of his duty can appear to be in conflict with his professional values of respect for persons and client self-determination. Whilst recognizing this Brenda Hoggett argues that rather than 'a special breed of mental health policeman': 'How much better that it should be a trained social worker: he should be best equipped to persuade the patient to enter hospital informally if at all possible, to make an independent judgement about whether compulsion is necessary and above all to handle the admission with sympathy and common sense so that the patient and his family suffer as little as possible' (Hoggett 1976:14). To this can be added MIND's comment that social workers may well be the professional group most aware of local community support and action on behalf of mentally ill people (MIND 1976).

The British Association of Social Workers (BASW) goes further than Hoggett in arguing that a social worker is not only better than 'a special breed of mental health policeman' but better also than the patient's relatives in determining what is best for the mentally ill person (BASW 1977b).

While the duties of the social worker are made clear in the Act, his role appears to be regarded as being primarily administrative rather than professional, and it is not difficult to understand why BASW should argue strongly that this role should be more clearly identified as one which complements rather than merely implements that of the doctors. The basis for this argument is the claim to professional expertise that a social worker can bring to bear in assessing certain aspects of the situation: 'We see the social worker as having a particular understanding of family and social functioning which helps him to distinguish those elements of the patient's behaviour which arise from environmental tensions rather than from psychiatric disorder' (BASW 1977).

Social work training and experience is primarily in evaluation of the social setting and not in the diagnosis of mental illness. The law makes it quite clear that the medical grounds for admission are the exclusive province of the doctors, and the social worker cannot, therefore, oppose the diagnosis of the existence of mental disorder (Hoggett 1976; BASW 1977b). He does, however, have to be satisfied that an *application for admission* should be made after a medical recommendation of formal admission has been given. He is expected to make an independent evaluation of the situation which focuses not on the accuracy of the psychiatric opinion but on the environment of the patient, on his home, family, and surrounding community. He views all these in the context of his knowledge of the resources available to meet in the most appropriate way the needs that he and others identify. The achievement of a balanced solution between the possibly conflicting interests of the parties whom the social worker has an obligation to help and protect, requires the exercising of professional judgement as to how differing needs and demands can be reconciled or the most feasible satisfactory compromise can be reached. Such a judgement will depend on an assessment of the risks to which each party is or will be exposed; the danger to the mentally ill person and those around him resulting from observable and foreseeable hazards in the existing situation have to be weighed against the hazards of admission. Admission, whilst reducing or eliminating some dangers, might at the same time create new hazards to which all concerned will to some degree be exposed.

Before proceeding it should be explained why from this point the central figure in the admission situation is referred to as 'the patient' rather than 'the client'. The reasons have in fact already been explored above but have not been made explicit in this context. First, once the diagnosis of mental illness has been made the initial step in the medicalization of the problem, that is its placement within the medical model, has been taken and the conferring of the sick role on the mentally ill person has been effected; in this role the primary responsibility for the treatment of the illness has been accepted by the medical practitioners and the person suffering from it becomes their 'patient'. Second, given the duties of the social worker towards people other than the person manifesting signs of mental illness, it can be misleading and an over-simplification to imply that the primary focus of concern will necessarily be the mentally ill person by designating only him as 'the client'. A third reason is that the term 'patient' can conveniently be taken to refer to the person who has been diagnosed as mentally ill throughout the following discussion and thus obviates the need for clumsy repetition.

An important risk element in the admission of the mentally ill, particularly where the use of compulsion is involved, arises with the possibility that the patient will be unnecessarily deprived of his rights and liberty. This risk and the dangers associated with it have been the subject of much debate, and an attempt has been made to provide a prescriptive formula for minimizing them: 'No person should be admitted to a treatment facility unless a prior determination is made that the facility is the least restrictive setting necessary for that person' (Gostin 1975:142). But 'least restrictive setting' is a relative concept which defies legislative definition. It can, nevertheless, be meaningful at a localized level where the worker is sufficiently familiar with the range of facilities available to be able to make a comparative assessment of both the degree of restriction and the availability of appropriate treatment. A system of priorities, however, which gives precedence to the consideration of restriction rather than of the availability of treatment is one which a social worker might find of questionable value in application. Since the social worker, in this context, has no formal alternative to accepting the medical diagnosis, then it seems proper to argue that priority should be given to securing for the patient treatment which will alleviate his suffering as soon as possible. The law views the mental illness as the immediate source of danger because of the further hazards it creates and it is these that constitute the initial area of concern; the dangers associated with loss of liberty can be seen as emanating from and secondary to those more specifically associated with the mental illness. The social worker, therefore, has to attempt to reconcile the immediate needs of those involved with the anticipated possible long-term effects on the patient and others of the courses of action available.

Admission, as already stated elsewhere in this book, is often seen as, at best, the least unattractive alternative form of intervention. But it should never be seen as a totally negative exercise – if we are convinced that nobody will gain anything from admission, even when this might be in the apparently negative form of a reduction in loss or danger of loss, then there is no justification for pursuing it. The possible gains of admission should be as significant a consideration in assessment as the potential dangers of not admitting.

A danger, particularly perhaps in mental health work, is that decisions will be based more on the subjective anxieties of those making them than on an objective assessment of the need for treatment, containment, or protection. If this danger is to be reduced it is essential that the decision makers, including the social worker, have as BASW recommend: 'a basic knowledge of the nature and classification of mental disorders, of facilities for care and treatment, of relevant law and procedure, and of good professional practice in this field' (BASW 1977b:22). Under 'good professional practice' could be included the ability to recognize subjective needs and feelings and to disentangle them from those of others.

Having once established that the need for admission is not simply the 'easiest' or most expedient solution to a problem of disposal, and having identified the range of resources available offering appropriate care and treatment, the alternatives can then be considered in terms of the principle of 'least restrictive setting'. Again, the decision about which setting is the least restrictive will depend on what alternatives are available locally and on the decision maker's knowledge of them. This was recognized by David Ennals, then Secretary for Social Services, in an interview in December, 1978, on the recently published white paper on the review of the Mental Health Act: 'There is no objective measure or test that could be applied in decisions about appropriate placements. These are matters of professional judgement in the light of the individual circumstances of the case and the facilities that may be available locally. We have suggested that the social worker should have the responsibility to satisfy himself when making an application for compulsory admission that the care and treatment offered is in the least restrictive conditions practicable in all the circumstances' (Draper 1978).

It should be remembered that, as BASW implies in its questioning of the assumption of universal benevolence on the part of relatives, it cannot be taken for granted that the patient's home is the least restrictive environment nor, on the other hand, that a psychiatric hospital is the most. It should also be remembered that in mental health admissions generally the need for compulsion occurs relatively infrequently; to quote Clare (1976:337): 'Questions of responsibility do not arise in every case of mental illness. It is only in those mentally disturbed people who act out (or threaten to act out) their depressive, persecutory, or aggressive preoccupations that the degree and extent of their responsibility for their actions is queried.'

It emerges from what has been said so far that one of the most important and difficult tasks in which the social worker is involved in the admission situation is the attempt to achieve a balance between three crucial elements – society's concern for the treatment of mental illness, its concern with the liberty of the individual and its concern with its own protection. These elements are present in both the formal and the informal admission situations.

Informal admission requires first, that it is believed to be in the best interests of the patient and, second, that it is effected with his informed and voluntary consent. The patient should have freely chosen to be admitted. The reality of such a choice depends on the existence of alternatives, the patient's knowledge of them, and on his freedom from coercion – admission under the threat of compulsion is not voluntary.

A hazard to which an informal patient is exposed on admission, and about which he has a right to be informed, is that his legal status can be changed if in the opinion of the responsible medical officer such a change is thought to be necessary. As long ago as 1966 concern was being expressed that some informal patients only remained so for as long as they submitted to the decisions made about them by medical staff; as can possibly occur in admission, informal status was accepted by the patient only under the express or implied threat of compulsion. As this same report (Ministry of Health 1966) pointed out, an important consequence of informal status, coerced or otherwise, is that the patient is deprived of the right of appeal: 'In this way a patient may in theory be in hospital of his own volition, but in fact be under informal compulsion to remain there, and thus be bereft of the right to ask for the authority for his detention to be reviewed by the tribunal.' Although a formal patient is deprived of certain rights he does at the same time have procedural safeguards which are denied the informal patient; formal status, like admission itself, should not be seen as being entirely without benefit.

The intention of the Mental Health Act is that nobody should be formally admitted unless it has been previously established that he is unwilling to enter informally. This intention is in keeping with the report of the Percy Commission, on which the Act is largely based and of which one of the basic premises was that people suffering from mental disorder should, as far as possible, be treated in the same way as those suffering from physical illnesses and that compulsion and custody should be used as little as possible (DHSS 1978). The informal patient enters hospital on the advice of his doctor to receive the care and treatment he is advised is necessary or desirable. These are voluntary acts on his part and he has the right to leave the hospital should he so wish, and to decline to accept any course of treatment. But as the *Review of the Mental Health Act* observes all staff, whether in psychiatric or general hospitals, have a duty under common law to prevent patients coming to harm; for example they have a duty to prevent a confused patient from wandering if by doing so the patient would be putting himself or others at risk. The social worker should ensure that the patient is informed of these possible consequences of admission, the implications of his informal status, his rights and the duties of hospital staff, because they are all factors which he should have the opportunity to consider before deciding whether or not to accept the advice to enter hospital.

MIND has argued that formal admission should be resorted to only on the basis of behavioural criteria, on the degree of dangerousness which can be predicted from the observation of recent overt acts. In this way the use of compulsion would not be determined by medical criteria which assumes some underlying cause (illness) of which the behaviour is only a symptom, but by the recognition of phenomena apparent to and verifiable by non-medical observers. The other case in which MIND suggests compulsion would be justified is in a narrowly defined category of 'grave disablement' (Gostin 1975) where the individual requires to be admitted in his own best interests because of inability to provide for basic needs or to sustain life. It is argued that preventive confinement of a person because he *might* commit a dangerous act is improper in English law and yet it occurs in the case of the mentally disordered. A patient should only be formally admitted to a psychiatric hospital if evidence can be produced of mental disorder as a result of which he lacks appreciation of his own condition and dangerous propensities, and further, that he is admitted only if treatment is available which can alleviate his condition or strengthen his ability to regulate his behaviour.

In putting forward these arguments MIND would appear to be supporting the view that 'the institutional psychiatrist's primary function is as an agent of social defence, one who ensures that he employs his scientific expertise to protect society from the irrationally deviant, and the irrationally deviant from themselves' (Fennell 1977). It is difficult to see why the criteria for compulsory admission suggested by MIND should inspire any more confidence in their predictive reliability than the medical criteria endorsed by the Mental Health Act. Although the reliability of long-term psychiatric prognosis has frequently been questioned, there is evidence to show that psychiatric predictions in the short-term, crisis situation are a great deal more accurate (Monahan 1978). Reference to recent overt acts alone would seem to be a less adequate way of determining the degree of dangerousness in a situation than the viewing of those acts within the context of clinical evidence accumulated in the nosology of psychiatric practice and the prognoses for which it provides a base. In addition, it would appear to be inconsistent to devalue psychiatric assessment and at the same time to demand effective psychiatric treatment; the latter must to a great extent depend on the accuracy of the former.

It is arguable, therefore, that the criteria for compulsory admission suggested by MIND and endorsed by BASW in 'Mental Health Crisis Services — a new philosophy', offer no more effective means of reducing uncertainty in the realm of mental illness and civil liberties than those used in psychiatry. Indeed, an approach which emphasizes above all else the hazard posed by the loss of liberty could be seen as serving to increase the danger posed by the mental illness itself, because it undermines a most important objective of the Mental Health Act, namely that the doctors should be freed from legal encumbrances on the admission process in order to be able to help the patient at the earliest practicable stage in the development of his illness. Such an objective clearly rests on the belief that it is the mental illness itself which constitutes the greater danger and, because of the immediacy of the hazards it presents, demands priority over other considerations including that of the threat to civil liberty. It must also be based on an assumption of integrity and competence existing in the care and treatment of the mentally ill, but not an expectation of certainty in psychiatric diagnosis and prognosis; such an expectation would be as unreasonable of psychiatry as of any other branch of medicine.

The civil liberties approach to the mentally ill is, for some, disquieting. Kathleen Jones, for example, sees it as being retrograde in its emphasis on a legalistic view of procedures (Jones 1977). She points out that the 1959 Act was a conscious attempt to get away from over-rigid legal provisions which, framed by lawyers, prescribed exactly what a mental welfare officer should do in any conceivable circumstances and left nothing to his discretion; it sought to avoid the situation of piling safeguard on safeguard to protect the sane from illegal detention and thereby delaying certification and treatment until the person genuinely in need of care was obviously insane

(Jones 1972). In Jones' view the 1959 Act was 'an enabling act which freed practitioners and patients from the shackles of a highly legalistic system that labelled both the patients and the hospitals and prescribed special, often stigmatized procedures for them' (Jones 1977). She argues that progress and reform have involved minimizing the legal element in the care and treatment of mental disorder in favour of flexible procedures based on good training and common-sense decisions. The civil liberties approach is now threatening these reforms by focusing attention on the areas of compulsory admission and appeal procedures which affect only a small minority of the mentally ill. (As noted earlier, although formal admissions constitute a small minority of mental health admissions it is likely that they are disproportionately represented in those admissions involving social workers.)

It would seem that, depending on the point of view held, one of the most serious dangers to the mentally ill can result directly from the ideological position taken by those called upon to intervene in their lives. The works of Laing, Szasz, Cooper, Scheff, Clare and many others serve to indicate the wide variety of views taken and the intensity with which they can be promoted. Certainly, the perception of existing hazards and dangers in a given situation and the relative importance attached to them will be influenced to a very great extent by the convictions held about the nature of mental illness, its possible or probable causes and appropriate treatment. The way in which those hazards and dangers are dealt with by the social worker will be further determined by the way in which he views his primary function as being either to facilitate early care and treatment, uphold individual liberty, or afford collective protection. These aspects of the social work task deserve careful thought. The social worker has a great deal of discretion in how he fulfils the duties laid upon him by the Mental Health Act which, if anything, adds to the burden of responsibility he carries. Although he must be authorized by his employing authority to legitimately function as a mental welfare officer, legal responsibility for what he does is placed directly upon him as an individual and not as a representative of the local authority. Unlike his predecessor, the duly authorized officer, the social worker is no longer subject to the instructions of a magistrate but has, in fact, taken on some of the functions relating to the protection of the interests and liberty of the individual previously performed by a magistrate.

All these considerations serve to underline the seriousness of admission and of the social work role in the process of decision making. It is often not an easy role to fulfil, as BASW acknowledges: 'The social worker is usually, nowadays, a comparatively junior member of a large hierarchical department, and the independent status conferred upon him by the law is often difficult to sustain in practice' (BASW 1977b:23). Nevertheless, although the social worker cannot act without medical recommendations he is not bound by them; the decision to act on them or not is his and his alone and it is not one to be taken lightly. It calls for a high degree of professional judgement exercised on the basis of the skills and knowledge which BASW, in the quotation given above, recommend as basic requirements for the social worker dealing with the mentally ill and their problems.

THE ADMISSION PROCESS

Admission to a psychiatric hospital is likely to be a traumatic experience, a stressful and profoundly important event for all concerned. It is the consequence of a recognized crisis situation; a situation, that is, in which it has been recognized that usual means of coping have proved unequal or inappropriate to the task and that personal, familial, and wider environmental support structures have to be supplemented or replaced by the provision of an alternative environment offering special facilities.

Crisis theory (Parad 1965), which has assumed some prominence in social work, suggests that a crisis can be experienced in three different ways, as a threat, a loss, or as a challenge. If perceived primarily as a threat the main response will be anxiety, if seen as a loss the response will be depression, if the crisis is seen as a challenge the response will take the form of a mobilization of energy and resources directed towards finding ways of resolving the situation. There are elements in the mental health admission which can readily be seen as threats or losses; those elements which have the more positive characteristics of a challenge are less apparent but, hopefully, can in most cases be identified and used to offset the other two. An important aspect of the social work function could be the minimization of threat and loss and the maximization of the element of challenge with its connotations of potential gains.

The threat and loss factors in the mental health admission situation can have a cumulative effect. For both the patient and his family admission is an obviously disruptive experience in the normal pattern of life with largely unknown consequences. Ignorance and misconceptions might serve to increase any anxiety already created by preceding events. The patient is going to be subjected to change both of his physical environment and social role and both of these might arouse concern as to what is expected of him and what he can expect from others. For his family his removal will perhaps create a breach in its unity which will be experienced as a loss and, as in bereavement, evoke feelings of grief and despair.

An additional consideration is the degree to which the mental illness impairs the patient's ability to appreciate what is happening around him, or distorts his perception of what is going on and what is said about or to him. If compulsion is used it might be a realization of one of the patient's most intense fears, loss of control and responsibility for what happens to him.

Bowlby (1973) has referred to the cumulative nature of fear-stimulating situations, how the intensity of anxiety aroused by one event can be multiplied by the simultaneous occurrence of others. In the mental health admission some of these cumulative anxiety-provoking factors might be identified as: the initial anxiety which results in the original appeal for intervention; the confirmation that mental illness exists; the decision to advise admission and what this portends; the use of compulsion to enforce the decision if necessary, the admission or transfer process itself. All of these can contribute to an escalation of the level of anxiety and to an increase in the vulnerability of the patient and his relatives to harm. They can be further exacerbated by fear produced by lack of knowledge of what is happening and why, and where it might lead. The social worker, if he is aware of the possibility of these hazards existing, will seek to mitigate them and thereby diminish the dangers of loss, damage, or reduction of well-being to which those at the centre of the crisis situation can be exposed.

Admission, then, can be seen as a supervening crisis additional to that which resulted in intervention. In the decision-making stage it is the dangers associated with the mental illness which are the focus of attention; in the admission stage it is the hazards of the admission itself which become of immediate concern. Admission is a crisis created by those who having assessed the situation have decided that the hazards of admission are less than those associated with leaving the patient where he is. An important argument of this chapter, indeed one of the most important arguments of this book, is that the significance of this crisis and the necessity for it to be dealt with properly are no less than those of the events which lead up to the decision to admit; the same degree of competence and care on the part of the social worker is necessary as was required by the process of assessment and decision.

Once the decision to advise admission is made the social worker will wish to ensure that the patient and his family are informed and given the opportunity to talk about it. The degree of anxiety and distress might be high, making the absorbing of information difficult, but with patience and sensitivity the social worker can attempt to inform the patient of his rights, of the implications of admission and how it is to be effected. Such information might dispel at least some of the anxiety by decreasing feelings of helpless ignorance. It is essential, however, that in an attempt to reduce anxiety the social worker does not resort to prevarication or deceit; such methods can produce false hopes and expectations which might calm the situation in the short term but undermine the possibility of a future trusting relationship between the patient and his family and those claiming to be concerned with their interests. Apart from such practical concerns, to deliberately mislead, for whatever motive, is irreconcilable with the basic social work value of respect for persons.

The giving of information is an essential part of the first of the four stages into which the admission process can be divided – preparation, separation, transition, and incorporation. Preparation can also include explanation of the reasons why admission is thought to be appropriate. It would certainly include information about where the patient is going and how he is going to get there. It would extend to listening to the patient's family and answering their queries. In some cases it will involve giving reassurance about practical matters and taking any steps necessary to safeguard interests threatened by admission, e.g. ensuring that property will remain secure or pets properly cared for.

In the case of compulsory admission it is customarily the social worker who ensures that the appropriate documents are correctly completed and arranges for the patient's transfer. The Mental Health Act specifies certain periods of time within which, following the completion of formalities, admission can be effected. Oram (1978) in one of the few attempts in social work literature to examine mental health admission procedures in practice enquiries:

> 'How did the legislators intend that we should use this time? Did they visualise a long and difficult process of flight, hide, search and capture? Or did they anticipate levels of care which would use some of the time first to reconcile the patient to the idea of admission, and secondly, to influence family relationships so that they could prepare for admission in an atmosphere where the trauma was not substantially different from that surrounding other types of illness?'

It would seem to be the latter view which is most in keeping with the Act's intention to diminish the differences in the ways in which mental illness and other forms of illness are perceived and, in that case, the time periods provided in the Act can be seen as breathing spaces which offer the social worker the opportunity to seek ways of reducing the danger of the admission situation, by ameliorating some of the threat and loss hazards which produce it. It is a time during which areas of uncertainty can be clarified and the patient and his family can be allowed to further explore their anxieties and to reconcile themselves to the necessity for admission and the potential advantages to be gained from it.

Oram comments that usual practice, however, would seem to be that, irrespective of which section of the Act is being used, the patient is removed to hospital as soon as the necessary documentation and transport arrangements have been completed. He suggests that there is a widespread assumption that the use of compulsion *necessarily* implies an emergency situation. Whilst this might be true in many cases where the need for treatment and/or containment is immediate, it is not true of all formal admissions. It is for the social worker to assess whether the possible advantages of postponing admission outweigh the hazards.

Another mistaken assumption which Oram suggests is often made is that emergency implies compulsion, that is that unwillingness is an inevitable corollary of acute mental illness and that if, for whatever reason, consent is not clearly expressed compulsory powers are justified. In fact, informal status is not intended to be confined only to the patient who is 'voluntary' in the sense of actively wishing to accept the advice to enter hospital, it extends also to those who are *not actively unwilling*. This principle is restated in the *Review of the Mental Health Act*: 'Where the patient does not have the mental capacity to know what is taking place an absence of objection on his part cannot be taken either as implying or withholding consent to admission' (DHSS 1978). In Oram's view, however, 'the concept of emergency is still inextricably associated with the need for compulsion, so that doctors and social workers sometimes overlook the consideration of whether the patient is actually unwilling and some hospitals make compulsory procedures a condition of admission when crises occur outside normal hours'.

Regarding these two, often inappropriate assumptions, that compulsion necessarily implies emergency and that emergency necessarily implies compulsion, Oram concludes:

'The anticipation of adverse reaction is so great that a state of emergency exists regardless of the mode of admission. In addition, the stances adopted to counteract reaction often become a self-fulfilling prophecy that provokes the behaviour it is intended to prevent and which may be quoted to justify both the use of compulsion and the unseemly haste.'

If Oram is correct in believing that such responses occur in many mental health admissions, we must conclude that social workers are in practice often contributing to precisely the sort of escalation of tension in the situation which this chapter argues it should be one of their primary aims to reduce.

Oram's concern that these responses indicate a high degree of anxiety in the social worker and/or an outdated view of mental illness is perhaps similar to that of the BASW Mental Health Committee as reflected in the quotation given above outlining the basic requirements of approved mental health social workers. It is not that social workers are any more likely than family doctors, policemen, relatives, and others who might be involved to be anxious or hold outdated views or react inappropriately, but that the nature of their professional role demands that they should ensure as far as possible that they do not. If such factors are not considered a situation of danger can be artificially generated in which unnecessary haste can provoke in the frightened, confused, and uninformed patient precisely the sort of response which justifies compulsion and emergency action.

The presumption of urgency and unwillingness perhaps partially accounts for the fact that in some areas of the country 80 per cent of formal admissions are under Section 29, and why some hospitals will not accept informal patients out of normal hours (DHSS 1978; BASW 1977). It need hardly be added that a social worker would never feel, or be, justified in making an application for compulsory or emergency admission merely on the grounds of administrative expediency or convenience.

Preparation, the first stage of admission, will inevitably involve consideration of the second stage, separation. For the patient and his family separation will be both a physical and an emotional fact, and how negatively this will be experienced is likely to be affected by a number of factors. Amongst these might be included the nature of immediately preceding events (including the preparatory work carried out), the quality of existing relationships, expectations of the outcome of admission and the degree to which each person has become resigned to the need for admission. Separation can render the patient and his family vulnerable to feelings of being rejected or rejecting, of being abandoned or abandoning, to feelings of inadequacy, guilt, shame, and to a sense of loss and its corollary, grief. As with any experience of grief it is important that its expression is not stifled or denied (Parad 1965; Parkes 1975). The social worker should be able to allow the ventilation of anxious and sorrowful feelings if they are present and not attempt to smother them with denial or false reassurance. The need is not to encourage expression of these feelings but to facilitate it by being attentive, concerned, and patient, by answering questions forthrightly and providing information freely. Lindemann (1976) states four things to be avoided by all helping professionals in work with grieving patients following bereavement which can usefully be applied to the separation stage of admission:

(1) administering questionnaires or firing questions;
(2) bringing up emotionally charged topics that the patient should not even think about at that time;
(3) expecting instant communication;
(4) running away after receiving a significant piece of information.

Transition begins in a psychological sense as soon as those involved become properly aware of the decision to admit; in a physical sense it is the stage of actual movement from one place to another. For the patient it involves the leaving of the familiar for the relatively, or completely unknown. How he perceives this removal will largely depend on what has taken place beforehand and on the amount of trust he has in those who are advising or directing him. It will depend also on the expectations he has of the outcome of admission and his preconceptions of the nature of his new role as patient and the consequences of it.

In the case of formal admissions the duty for effecting the removal of the patient to hospital is laid upon the social worker. This does not mean that the social worker is necessarily expected to physically accompany the patient, but considering the crucial importance of the role of the social worker in the preceding decision-making process and preparation work, good practice might seem to indicate that he should. One argument supporting this, as Bowlby has noted, is the immense difference created in the intensity of anxiety aroused in a situation by the presence or absence of a familiar person. Another argument might be the fourth point quoted from Lindemann's study; the social worker is likely to have been given a good deal of significant information on which to base his decision and not to implement that decision himself might be perceived by all involved as 'running away' or betrayal of their confidence. There is often no good reason why a relative should not also accompany the patient. This might offer valuable reassurance to both the patient and his family and help to alleviate some of the distress of separation by providing a familiar link between home and hospital.

The last stage of admission is incorporation – the integration of the patient within the treatment setting. A unique aspect of the mental health admission from the social work point of view is that once the patient is accepted by the hospital the social worker loses any formal control over what might happen to him – the client is no longer only a designated patient, he is in the environment specifically designed to accommodate him in his new role. Once he enters the hospital he comes directly under the care of medical and nursing staff, and matters such as treatment and discharge are the concern of hospital staff, relatives, and Mental Health Review Tribunals, areas upon which the social worker can exercise only limited and informal influence.

This situation is quite different to that of admitting, for example, a child to a children's home or an elderly person to residential accommodation. In these situations the staff of the establishments will be employed by the same authority that employs the field social worker and finances the institution; and more importantly, both residential and field work staff can be expected to perceive problems and priorities of care and treatment and ultimate objectives in similar ways, and to agree on approaches taken to these aspects of client need. In other words, field work and residential social work have a great deal in common in addition to their undoubted differences.

This common ground shared by different social work settings can provide a continuity for social work practice which is unlikely to be as easy in the case of the mentally ill admitted to a psychiatric hospital. The risks, hazards, and dangers to which the patient will be subject once he has entered hospital are beyond the social worker's control; this should be an important factor to consider in the decision-making process. If the social worker has carefully assessed the situation, made what he believes to be a proper decision and has consistently applied his knowledge and skills in the service of those he is there to help and protect, there is little more that can be expected of him regarding the admission process.

A question which remains is: when, for the social worker, does the admission process end? The answer might well be determined by people other than the social worker. It is possible, even probable, that he will be unable to follow the process through to what he considers from a social work point of view to be a satisfactory conclusion. Hospital practice might dictate that he leaves 'his client/their patient' and his belongings at the reception desk or he might be turned away at the entrance to the ward. Possibly this is as it should be, but, on the other hand, the social worker might feel that having been with the patient throughout what has been a difficult, if not harrowing, experience it would be inappropriate to quit him without attempting to achieve some overlapping of the ante and post admission phases. He might wish that the delivery of the patient into the care of the hospital should not be an abrupt exchange but a carefully paced transfer. One way in which this might be achieved could be by accompanying the patient to the ward, introducing him to nursing staff, and remaining until he is seen by the duty doctor, or has found a seat in the lounge; until, in fact, he has had an opportunity to orientate himself, albeit in a limited way, to his new surroundings.

The question of follow-up is not strictly within the area of discussion of this chapter but some observations are appropriate here because of the way in which they might influence attitudes to the admission process. Duty rotas, and the organization of intake teams and emergency teams can often make further contact with the patient difficult. Follow-up by the social worker who has participated in the admission might be seen as impracticable, inappropriate, or bureaucratically undesirable. Whilst it is possible to appreciate the reasons why this should be so, not least those relating to efficiency, it is not a situation that all social workers might accept without unease.

The reason for this unease would be the conviction that underlying and guiding the social worker's actions throughout the assessment, decision making, and admission processes would be his concern with the individual welfare of all concerned. This concern would manifest itself in a caring attitude towards each person that would not be confined to the present but would seek to ease the problems of the here and now at minimum cost in short- and long-term individual well-being. Medicine's primary concern is with what the person 'has' – his illness, the law's main concern is with what he does; basic to social work practice is the profession's overriding concern with what a person is. It is for this reason that whilst the task of ensuring that a problem is dealt with as efficiently as possible is a necessary part of the social worker's role it is not sufficient. In being involved in the admission he has used his professional skills to calculate the relative seriousness of numerous dangers to which the mentally ill person and others are exposed; whatever his decision it is extremely unlikely that it will eliminate all dangers, and quite likely that it will have unavoidably created new ones. His commitment to the welfare of those in whose interests he has acted extends beyond the immediate situation and, in consequence, he does not absolve himself of all responsibility for what happens to them subsequently in a situation which his decision has significantly influenced. His professional task, therefore, does not, according to this view, end with the delivery of the patient to hospital. It would be argued that despite the requirements of efficiency, the social worker who has shared the important experience of admission with the patient and his family should do so in anticipation of continuing a relationship with them which will be founded on the relationship made during this shared experience. In this way the possibility of admission becoming merely a routine, standardized procedure to be accomplished with the minimum of trouble is less likely to occur, and admission will continue to demand the same amount of attention to individual need and the same importance will be placed on the development of positive relationships as in any other sphere of social work practice.

This would imply that while the admitting social worker would not necessarily assume long-term responsibility for the case, he would see the patient at least once after admission; maybe to introduce the social worker who will maintain future contact and to discuss future plans, or merely to ascertain that the need for continued social work involvement does not exist. It would also mean that the admitting social worker would ensure, once the admission itself has been completed, that the family has no immediate problems that have been neglected and would offer them a further opportunity to ventilate their feelings about what has occurred and to give them any information they require, for example such basic facts as the ward to which the patient has been admitted, the name of his consultant, the hospital telephone number, and so on. If the need for further contact is expressed the social worker should be able to give the assurance that he will provide it, if only by again extending the continuity to the point of introducing a replacement.

In conclusion, one point about mental health admissions which has been neglected here should be recognized. For some, perhaps more than we often realize, admission to a psychiatric hospital might represent relief from what has become intolerable stress. For the patient admission can offer the hope of treatment and recovery and the promise of asylum from the

demands of day-to-day life which have grown increasingly difficult to meet. His family might see the hospital as a refuge where
he can be restored to his usual level of functioning in a purpose-
fully therapeutic environment whose main function is to return
him to normal life as soon as possible. The components of
protection, support, containment, and treatment offered by a
hospital are all prospective gains from admission. Whether
these prospective gains outweigh the hazards and dangers
involved in the admission process and its consequences is one of
the most important and difficult decisions a social worker is
called upon to make, from his own point of view, but even more
so from his clients'.

7 Admission and the Elderly

Paul Brearley

Discussions of social work with the elderly have ranged from the gloomily descriptive, through the dismally prophetic, to the euphorically evangelical. The following quotations, the first written in 1955, and the second in 1978 are fairly typical:

> 'To effect change in the public attitude toward old age will require the work of many forces. The need for new social interventions must be met by an inter-disciplinary approach in which each profession will be called upon increasingly to make its contribution. The prospects for success have never been more encouraging' (Greenleigh 1955).

> 'It is hardly possible to feel proud of the way society has treated the elderly over the last twenty years. We have increasingly forced them into a separate world, in terms of standards of comfort in the home, standards of living, and of housing . . . We are now in one of those periods in which many people think that the elderly should have less priority than other groups and that the problem of old age has been solved. The evidence suggests that such solutions are often far off indeed' (Bosanquet 1978).

Over twenty years separates the two comments and although there does not seem to be any reason to accept that the elderly are materially worse off than they were twenty years ago, in relative terms their circumstances may have improved less than those of younger people. It continues to be argued, moreover, that the solutions that are available to the problems experienced by old people are inadequate and it is sometimes hard to believe that we have progressed very far in any direction in our provision of services for the elderly. This is, of course, not so: many changes have taken place. In part this is the result of the increase in the numbers of very old people which has become so evident. Moroney (1976) suggests that if current population projections hold over the next thirty years there will be almost three-quarters of a million more old people of whom 88 per cent will be over the age of seventy-four and 41 per cent will be over eighty-four. Other changes in services have been linked to changes in the organization of social services delivery.

The pressures on services have changed but the basic concepts of good social work practice remain much the same. It is inevitable that the altered organizational context of practice affects the ways in which these basic concepts can be followed through. Several years ago I contributed a paper to *Social Work Today* (Brearley 1972) which was intended to highlight the problems involved in the system, which many social work departments used, of maintaining long waiting lists for old people's homes. Waiting lists seemed to be used as a way of avoiding taking action: the problem which is put on a waiting list is a problem out of the way. Since that time it seems that the primary difficulty has become, in one sense, the reverse of this: that many old people no longer have time to wait for admission to care. The increase in emergency admissions (DHSS 1976c) means that more and more of those admitted are given no time to prepare. The feature of social work and the elderly which has grown so much in importance is embodied in the elements of haste, of urgency, and of emergency and in the nature of risk, vulnerability, and protection. The interrelationships of these words and their careless and haphazard use have important implications for the understanding of good practice. This chapter will consider very briefly some of the available perspectives on ageing and old age, in social work, and will describe the hazards of old age before discussing the specific hazards and potentials of admission to care for old people.

KEY CONCEPTS IN SOCIAL WORK AND THE ELDERLY

It is difficult to explore admission without a detailed background explanation of perspectives on ageing. Unfortunately space does not permit this but background reading can be found in a number of sources. Elder (1977) has written passionately about the position of older people in a book written when she was herself old and similarly Gibberd (1977), Fry (1954), and Davies (1975) give a picture of what ageing is like from the perspective of older people themselves. I have written elsewhere about relevant theoretical and research perspectives on old age (Brearley 1975, 1976b, 1977).

Against the background of these detailed perspectives some of the central issues for social work practice can be considered. Much of the important material can be found in the British Association of Social Workers guidelines (BASW 1977a) which briefly discuss the need for knowledge and for changes in attitudes at all levels of society as well as within the profession. The breadth of ground which is relevant to the subject is too great to cover fully but some concepts are repeated in much of the social work literature and a discussion of these will point to further reading.

(i) Loss and Transition

There have been two general approaches to the discussion of social work and ageing. One approach has focused on the problems experienced by older people in material and emotional terms. They are said to lose choice, family, friends, and money; their health deteriorates along with their general physical abilities, and their environment is no longer adequate for their needs. The alternative approach has taken a developmental view of ageing, suggesting that old people are engaged in a progression of life and that the solutions to their problems should aim to restore them to a normal process of ageing.

It is clear that social workers are primarily engaged in providing basic, practical services for old people (whether this *should* be so is a matter for debate). An important study in Southampton (Goldberg *et al.* 1977) found that 84 per cent of elderly and physically disabled clients referred to an Area Social Services Office received some form of practical help. It is also clear that elderly clients are more likely to feel satisfied with the service they receive than younger clients are.

The evidence suggests, then, that the elderly receive – and are pleased to receive – mainly practical help from Social Services.

(ii) Satisfaction and Adaptation

The fact that elderly clients show more satisfaction than younger ones do is perhaps not surprising. Other studies have shown that older people are generally more likely to express satisfaction. A recent study (Age Concern 1977a) found that the elderly rated their overall satisfaction with life higher than did younger people – in spite of various objectively adverse circumstances. However, about one fifth of the elderly subjects in this study expressed very low levels of satisfaction, not only with their life as a whole but also with all the other aspects of life studied except for their health.

The evidence also suggests that although the majority of old people lead satisfied lives, there is a substantial minority of people who are very unhappy.

(iii) Dependence and Interdependence

One of the main factors underlying demand for Social Services by the elderly is the availability – or non-availability – of supporting friends or family. If old people need help it is several times more likely to be obtained from their spouse, children, or other relatives, than from Social Services: in personal care tasks, relatives are nearly always more important than health or social workers, and elderly people prefer to take their worries to relatives (Age Concern 1974). In Abrams' study of over-75s (1978) when respondents were asked to give their own descriptions of what makes for a satisfying life for people like themselves the biggest single group of replies was in terms of 'having good neighbours and good friends' and this was particularly true of those living alone.

Studies have consistently shown that the elderly as a group

are closely integrated into their communities by the things they do for others and have done for them in return. There remains, however, the minority – particularly the very old – who have few, or no supporting people and who make the greatest demands on Social Services. As Professor Olive Stevenson (1978b) has suggested 'we must commit ourselves to maintaining family ties through support to relatives, forming a partnership between the family and the wider society'.

Social work with old people has always been and will always be concerned with these elements. The importance of loss and transition, and of dependence – and most of all of *Interdependence* must be fundamental but their expression is closely influenced by the pressures of demand and by resources. At the present time it is becoming increasingly obvious that they should be seen in relation to the risk component.

(iv) Risk: Freedom and Safety

It has been widely argued that the very elderly infirm and disabled need access to a range of medical, residential, welfare, domiciliary, and other services so that they can exercise some degree of choice in the kind of care they receive (Age Concern 1975). This assumption rests on a value-judgement, expressed by Malcolm Johnson (1976) as the belief that older people are entitled to select their own destiny, within given limits. It is this final qualification – 'within given limits' – which may present the practitioner with the greatest difficulty. While it is not difficult to secure agreement on the right of old people to freely choose the kind of life they wish to lead it is less easy to define the limits of that freedom. The freedom of an old lady to choose to live in her own home, for instance, may depend upon the willingness of a neighbour to continue caring for her: one problem may be that the free choice of one person curtails that of another. A further problem arises when the old lady's choice to stay at home exposes her to considerable danger: the social worker may have to decide whether (in the extreme situation) to compel her to move to the comparative physical safety of an old people's home or to leave her to face probable danger alone. As was discussed in Chapter 2 the balance of safety and freedom involves risk-taking and risk-bearing.

The hazards and dangers to which old people are exposed are being increasingly carefully investigated. In the planning context it is now possible to identify certain predictive factors within a given population and to plan for additional services which Hall suggests will be necessary where:

'(1) the elderly population is above the national average;
(2) the over-75 population is above the national average;
(3) the over-85 population is above the national average;
(4) the elderly population has large numbers in social classes IV and V;
(5) the elderly population has large numbers living alone;
(6) a high proportion of the elderly population is in sub-standard housing; and
(7) a large proportion of families are unable or unwilling to provide support for the elderly e.g. where the area provides good work opportunities for women' (Hall, MacLennan, and Lye 1978:23).

Exposure of individuals to these factors does not necessarily mean that they are in urgent need. As was suggested earlier the subjective meaning of the situation to the individual is as important as an objective appraisal. Housing may be 'sub-standard' in comparative terms but to someone who has lived there for sixty years it feels familiar, and safe. Living alone is not, of itself, a problem but it predisposes to loneliness which can be a problem. In a review of research studies on domiciliary care (Goldberg and Connelly 1978) it was pointed out that although there was a general relationship between the amount of Home Help hours allocated and tasks to be done, help allocated did not clearly match 'needs' as indicated by the person's capacity and circumstances. What seems of particular importance is the precipitating factor in any individual situation in terms principally of the subjective perception by the old person that he has a problem. Some of the most important specific hazards can be identified.

(1) Most important to the elderly are the hazards to basic survival needs. The threats to physiological survival in terms particularly of lack of food and warmth have been identified. (a) Malnutrition is not common in Britain and surveys have shown that the food intake of the elderly is, on the whole, adequate (Stanton and Exton Smith 1970). The small proportion of the population who are malnourished are likely to be those who are disabled, housebound, and isolated (Brocklehurst 1978). (b) A study of hypothermia by Wicks (1978) has shown that large proportions of elderly people have cold living conditions and suggests that several tens of thousands of people over 65 at the time of the survey had hypothermia, within the terms of his definition. Although these figures are somewhat speculative the danger is clearly an important one. (c) A government survey, published in 1978 has shown that there is a marked decline in income level with age; and that (d) in respect of virtually all important housing amenities households where the head is aged 85 or over are worse off (Hunt 1978).

(2) Hazards to health are also of primary importance: studies have consistently shown the close relationship between health and satisfaction in the elderly.

(3) Mental impairment is a major feature of old age. Severe psychiatric illnesses have been found in some 10 per cent of all people over 65, and this proportion has been said to rise to 60 per cent in those with persistent physical ill health (Post 1974). Brain failure is particularly important: it has been estimated that in the United Kingdom about 13 per cent of those over 75 have a significant degree of brain failure and the proportion for those over 80 rises to 22 per cent (Hall, MacLennan, and Lye 1978).

(4) Bereavement and loneliness are common features of old age that contribute to breakdown. They have been linked through the use of the term 'desolation' (Shanas *et al.* 1968): living alone is not necessarily a problem and grief is a normal process with which most people cope within the family. When the isolated person is bereaved, however, it is likely that he (or more

probably she) will become depressed and lonely – or desolated.

This list is not exhaustive: there are many factors which make life hazardous for individuals. An important role for the social worker is the identification and evaluation of the hazards and dangers with the old person: an assessment of a risky or problem situation can only be made in association with the central person – the elderly client. This assessment is made in the light of knowledge about the resources that are available. For many old people the solution will be found in provision of services at home and this aspect is fully discussed in the following chapter. For a minority of old people – and it should be remembered that the majority of the elderly continue to lead an integrated life in their own home and community – residential care may prove to be the most appropriate answer. Before reaching this decision, however, the hazards of admission to institutional care should be taken into account.

REASONS FOR ADMISSION

Residential facilities for the elderly are used principally as a risk-management resource. Local authority priority grading systems are frequently based explicitly on the risk concept. The system in use in Coventry in 1976, for example, includes the following gradings:

'AA is the highest priority grade accorded where there is a high and continuing risk factor in the social situation despite the maximum possible input of fieldwork and domiciliary services . . .

A grade covers similar circumstances but here the risk factor is generally somewhat ameliorated by supportive help available to the client . . .

B covers those applications where a present risk factor is not apparent but there is clearly an unsatisfactory living situation' (Quoted in DHSS 1976a).

A DHSS survey (1976c) suggests that careful assessment of elderly applicants is often not possible because many requests for admission present themselves as emergencies: in one large county it was estimated that 40 – 50 per cent of admissions presented themselves as emergencies. The report shows that, although preparation for admission was recognized to be necessary the process was short circuited by the need for emergency admission. In these circumstances it is inevitable that people coming into care often do so at an advanced stage of physical, mental, or social deterioration. Any discussion of admission procedures and practices must take due account of these factors.

A study of two hundred admissions to a large residential home in Edinburgh (Lowther and McLeod 1974) found that half were over the age of 80; a large majority were widowed, single, or separated; a quarter came from hospital and half from home with the rest coming from other homes or hostels. Seventy five per cent of people admitted had some functional impairment and the authors of the study suggest that disability was a major factor leading to admission. A smaller study in the East Riding of Yorkshire (Cigno 1979) of thirty-seven residents in a purpose-built home found an average age of 83 years. A quarter of residents had been incontinent on admission and another quarter were considered confused: following admission twenty-one residents deteriorated, ten showed no change, and six improved. Two main groups of admissions were suggested: those who 'needed virtually nursing care' and a smaller number of homeless elderly for whom there was no alternative residence.

Moroney (1976) quotes four studies which, over the last fifteen years, have identified similar reasons why people seek admission to care. The main reason given is an inability of the person to look after him, or herself, or an anticipated inability to do so in the future. Admission is often preceded, and perhaps precipitated by an illness or the death of a family member who provided care. Loneliness, and family stress seem to account for a relatively small proportion of applications – each less than 10 per cent.

The picture that emerges suggests that the majority are very old, physically and mentally frail, and socially unsupported applicants who are frequently unable to obtain admission except in emergency. This emphasis on emergency may be a result of the fact that some do not ask for help until they are forced to do so or it may be because resources are so limited that only those who are in the greatest – most imminent and serious – danger receive help. It may also be to some extent that preventive social work practice is less effective than it could be. Whatever the reasons the haste with which a large proportion of old people are admitted is a problem. Older people tend to be slower and they do need more cues and information before they are willing to make a decision and take action. The social worker will be concerned with balancing the individual old person's need for time to think and prepare, against the pressing physical needs for care, warmth, food, or support. The necessary skill lies in being able to take the pressure from the old person during the process of deciding to apply. The priority is therefore to identify the sources of pressure – the hazards: it will often be possible to provide substitute supports on a short-term basis to give some breathing space.

Not all old people are admitted as emergencies of course and it has often been suggested that a proportion of admissions are unnecessary, even in the context of the limited resources available. A hundred old people in Manchester, for example, were screened at the time of their acceptance for residential care and it was found that alternative care was more appropriate in thirty-two of the cases (Brocklehurst *et al.* 1978). It does seem likely that some people enter care without there being a full consideration of the options. The proportion doing so, however, will almost certainly vary with prevailing local conditions, and available resources.

A sizeable group of admissions to residential care come from hospital, or from other homes. The administrative divisions between health and social services have led to the unfortunate practice of body-swapping, whereby a sick resident can only be transferred to hospital in exchange for a patient from the hospital. This has meant that there has been little time for preparation for the actual transfer and in some of the larger county areas some people have been admitted to homes many miles from their own home area and friends. A DHSS memorandum of guidance has now suggested that since most elderly patients admitted to hospital are discharged within three months, a resident's place in the old people's home should be retained for about three months. The memorandum also advises that the place could be used during that period, for short-term care (DHSS/Welsh Office 1977).

Short-term care is now recognized as an important way of giving relief to relatives looking after old people at home and authorities are increasingly making such provision. In such situations it is important that the nature and length of the stay should be clearly agreed: if relatives refuse to take the old person back home at the end of the stay this can only cause distress for all concerned. One answer to the problem is increased family support to prevent them from reaching a hopeless, and therefore desperate position. Two weeks short-term care each year may be enough for some families, but for others it may only serve to make them more aware of the burden they carry.

THE EXPERIENCE OF ADMISSION

If admission is inevitable then, as far as possible, the old person should be involved in discussion of the decision. This will not always be possible because some will be too confused to understand the reasons but only in acute emergency should lack of time prevent full discussion. One survey (Shaw and Walton 1978) concluded that about half of those being admitted to homes knew nothing about them before arrival. If preparation is based on imagination rather than realistic discussion and observation it is hardly surprising that some people feel abandoned and depressed after admission.

Morton Lieberman has researched and published widely on the effects of admission to care on old people over many years. In a book written with Tobin (1976) he identifies four explanations for the behaviours and responses observed over a period of admission. The first of these explanations relates to selection biases. Tobin and Lieberman found that there was a wide diversity of personality types present in the group admitted: no one type of person seeks admission to care. There is some support for this finding in studies in Britain (Pattie and Gilleard 1978) but it should be remembered that those coming into residential care are a particularly vulnerable group. They are, by operational definition, the group who are in greatest danger in the community and they bring a high degree of physical, intellectual, and emotional danger with them. It might be argued that those who come into residential care are those who are, in fact, the least likely to survive.

The second and most important finding of the Tobin and Lieberman survey relates to what they call the process effects before admission. 'The psychological portrait of the institutionalised older person who enters one of the better long-term care institutions is sketched in before the person actually enters and lives in the institutional environment' (p. 218). In other words, the psychological effects on the individual of institutional living which have been attributed to the effects of actually living in an institutional environment (Barton 1959) appear to be related more to reactions to the waiting period before admission. Tobin and Lieberman suggest that these effects are particularly attributable to 'the loss meaning of separation', and to the experience of being abandoned related to the dread of the impending event and to the expected separation. The relationships between those old people waiting for admission to care and those close to them are characterized by feelings of separation, rejection, and abandonment. Other studies have also confirmed the importance of the element of felt-rejection to adjustment following admission (Yawney and Slover 1973).

A third factor identified by Tobin and Lieberman is the effect of environmental discontinuity and they suggest that moving from one environment to another is associated with excess negative outcome and that effect is independent of the kind of environment, situation, or length of waiting period. The effect is particularly great in those who had lived transitionally in nursing homes, or who were more passive, or who had deteriorated physically.

Finally they suggest that even the best forms of institutional life for the elderly have harmful effects. In particular the new arrival is exposed to identification including 'being sick, being in need of care, being closer to death, and possessing a limited and uncontrollable future' (p. 220).

Other studies have also considered the effects of entering institutional living and these can be divided into those which have outlined the physical dangers and those which discuss psychological dangers. An early survey by Rosin (1966) suggests that 'admission of an old person to hospital entails a certain degree of risk'. In addition to the illness precipitating admission, complications may arise from the illness or indirectly from related factors, but also from factors already in the hospital, particularly infections. Entry to group living, then, exposes the elderly person to the physical stress of environmental change but also to existing infections among members of the group.

On the individual psychological level Litin (1956) has gone so far as to compare the reactions of the old person on admission to hospital with those of the child, emphasizing disorientation and anxiety. Others have discussed regression, rejection, and depression following admission (Kent 1963).

It has been extensively argued that relocation of the elderly is associated with negative outcomes – deterioration and early death. However the research suggests that a number of variables are important. The degree of change involved is a key factor: if there is limited change and the degree of disruption is minimized then the effects are less likely to be marked, and effective preparation and efficient transfer procedures can diminish the stress of the move (Gutman and Herbert 1976). A study in Britain (Pattie and Gilleard 1978) suggests that most elderly people are not necessarily affected by admission to care and the reported 'negative relocation effect' seems to be restricted to a small group of residents. For this group however the decrease in behavioural competence after admission is linked to 'increased vulnerability to the risk of mortality and of permanent hospitalisation in the following year'.

Much research has been devoted to identifying the type of person who is most vulnerable to the stress of moving. This research has been reviewed by Yawney and Slover (1973) who suggest that three groups of factors are important: the characteristics of the person moving, the preparations for the move, and the quality of the new environment. In relation to the first of these they identify organic brain damage; poor health or advanced degenerative physical changes; depression or the absence of hope. One of the most important factors is the person's usual coping pattern: if he has always been able to handle change then he is likely to make a good adjustment.

One study (Pablo 1977) which found that relocation had negative effects showed that these effects were minimized by '(a) careful planning of the move and the appreciable casework involved in the patient's preparation for relocation (b) the nature and degree of environmental change involved and (c) the voluntariness of the change involved'. Preparation has a measurable effect in reducing the stressful and potentially harmful effects of admission.

For the social worker, then, research suggests several factors of key importance for practice:

(1) those with a habitually passive approach to life are more vulnerable to negative outcome following admission;
(2) those who have a marked degree of brain failure, illness, or physical decline are also vulnerable;
(3) the *decision* to enter care is an important trigger to behavioural change. Withdrawn and self-centred behaviour is a feature of the waiting period as much as of institutional living;
(4) feeling abandoned, and separated are associated with negative outcome: felt-rejection is an important predictor;
(5) careful planning of the move and preparation of the old person can minimize stress and negative effects;
(6) Moving from one environment to another is, of itself, stressful and predictive of physical deterioration. This is particularly so of those who stay transitionally in nursing homes before final admission (this refers particularly to evidence from the USA where institutional definitions are rather different);
(7) the degree of change of environment is an important factor:

the more moderate the change the less marked the effect
may be;

(8) the quality of the new environment is influential in adjust·
ment to institutional living.

ADMISSION: THE FIELD WORKER'S ROLE

It has been pointed out in Chapter 3 that the concept of a 'right'
way of admitting someone to care is based on value assumptions. The justification for social work involvement in the
admission process — aside from the statutory and agency duties
and control of resources — stems from the fact that it is a
potentially stressful and damaging experience. The social
worker's role is concerned with the enhancement of well-being.
A further value assumption has also been proposed earlier in
this chapter, that older people have a right to be involved in
what is happening to them. It is important that things are done
not only to them, for them, and around them but also with
them.

The field worker's role is based, then, on a respect for human
dignity and the need to promote well-being. The understanding
and management of risk will, as has already been indicated, be
particularly concerned with uncertainty but also with assessing
likelihood and anticipating and evaluating outcomes. The social
worker will be involved in finding ways of anticipating what
may happen, and in reducing the uncertainty and therefore the
anxiety of the client, his family, and the worker himself.

A formal application for admission to an old people's home
should only be made when as assessment has been carried out
and when full discussions have taken place. It should be clearly
established that the hazards which make the current situation
undesirable cannot be removed or reduced. It should also be
clear that there are likely potential benefits to the move — if
only in the sense that the old person will not be in a worse
position after the move — and that the hazards of the move
itself can be minimized. Some families may try to put the social
worker into a collusive position, perhaps to avoid the pain and
distress of facing up to their inability to look after the elderly

relative. If the worker plays their game, filling in a form in another room and then persuading, or even tricking the old person into signing the form this can only build up problems for the future. Either the family will have to face the painful reality in the future, or their guilt and the old person's resentment may cause a permanent rift. Other families may try to bully the social worker into taking the action they want and try to avoid a consideration of the alternatives: there may be no real choice but this must be recognized through open discussion.

The decision that admission is the most suitable answer has to be made in the light of local resources. To make an application and then be placed on a long waiting list is frustrating and depressing, and as has been pointed out above, an extended period of waiting can be damaging: it can introduce rather than reduce danger. Once an application has been made admission should follow fairly soon and if this is not possible the client should receive a full explanation: to be kept waiting is hard enough but to be kept waiting and in uncertainty is un-acceptable and unnecessary. The social worker's next step is then to prepare the old person for leaving home in the right way. The actual move from the old environment to the new can be arranged in whatever is the most convenient and comfortable way. If the family are involved they should be encouraged and enabled to help but the social worker must judge each situation separately. The priority is to ensure that the old person is helped and supported through the anxiety and inevitable uncertainty of the admission.

An essential consideration at this time will be the protection of the people and property left behind. Some people do improve in residential care with food, warmth, and support and if they have sold their house and furniture may find themselves unable to escape. At a time when so many admissions are of very old and frail people it will be a very small proportion who do return home but nevertheless the possibility exists (Brearley 1977). The house and furniture should be preserved and protected in case the client wishes to return home, and this will at the very least give a feeling of security in the settling-in period. If the client wishes, however, arrangements should be made for the disposal of the property, with the client's full involvement. The property to be taken into the home should also be carefully discussed: the image that the old person presents when he first arrives at the home will be a lasting one – no-one entering a new situation wishes to take the wrong clothes, for example.

In order to reduce the objective uncertainty, and therefore the anxiety, the old person should be able to visit the home before admission. Sometimes it will be possible to arrange a trial short-stay, although pressures on the available resources make this a rare – if desirable – luxury. Some residential workers like to visit old people in their own homes before admission and some old people welcome this. This does give the new applicant a chance to present himself as someone with a past, with his own needs, and likes and dislikes but it will not always be possible or desirable. As in all social work with the elderly an individualized approach is necessary. A step-by-step approach to explaining and clarifying what is happening is essential in all cases. Meacher (1972) has described the way in which an old person, after being given little explanation of where she is going, may be taken by a social worker to a place she has never seen before. There is little wonder that when asked if she knows where she is the answer is confused: if no-one has told her she cannot answer. The problem arises when the label 'confused old person' is attached and she begins to be treated by others accordingly. The description may be a little extreme but it is uncomfortably familiar.

The field worker's role will be concerned with three main components:

(1) Making a careful assessment *with* the old person of all the alternatives. Admission should be considered as one alternative which, for most people, will only be chosen if there is no other option available. The first step is to identify the existing hazards, to consider whether they can be managed, and to balance the hazards of the status quo against those of the alternative courses of action.

(2) If admission to care is inevitable there should be full discussions and explanation with the old person and his family.

Practical issues of visiting the home, disposing of furniture etc. should be taken care of and adequate warning of the move must be given. Uncertainty will lead to anxiety and the worker will be concerned with helping with the anxiety but also with reducing the level of uncertainty: with giving information.

At this stage both worker and client are clearly taking and bearing risks and the nature of these risks need to be explored with the client.

(3) Sometimes emergency admission is unavoidable through fire, flood, illness of a member of the family, etc. If this is the case then preparation will be curtailed but it remains important to discuss the practicalities as well as the feelings involved with the old person both during and after admission. Some old people must be protected in their own interests. When a person is suffering from grave chronic disease, or is old, infirm, or physically incapacitated and is living in insanitary conditions and cannot care for himself, and is not receiving sufficient care from others the local authority may, on these grounds, apply to a magistrate's court for an order for the removal of the person to a suitable hospital (National Assistance Act, 1948: Section 47). Usually such an order will be for three months and must give a week's notice of removal, although emergency orders valid for three weeks can be made with immediate effect.

A sizeable proportion of admissions are from hospitals and it is important not to assume that this is simply an administrative procedure. To the old person it is as much a change as admission from home would be. Even if a swap of resident and patient has to be arranged the patient should be given several days notice of the move and should be given an opportunity to discuss the future. All property should be packed in front of the old person – and it is especially important that dentures, spectacles, and hearing aids are not forgotten. Continuity between the two environments can be provided by the field worker visiting beforehand and arranging the transfer and continuing to visit in the home, or by the residential social worker visiting in hospital before the move. It is also essential to give clear information to the family at this time.

ADMISSION: THE RESIDENTIAL WORKER'S ROLE

The Personal Social Services Council have begun to outline some of the main components of good practice in residential care (PSSC 1977). They suggest that the policy and objectives of the home should be clearly explained to the client and his family before entry and the policy on the taking of risks should also be explained so that it is clearly understood, particularly by the family. Written details about the home should be provided. If these approaches are adopted the objective uncertainty can be reduced. Similarly it is important to manage the subjective response to uncertainty – the anxiety – and on arrival the old person should be met by the officer-in-charge of the home and shown his room and introduced to some of the other residents. At this time the new arrival will experience a mixture of feelings: the fear of a new situation may be mixed with a feeling of relief at having reached sanctuary. The behaviour of the newcomer will take some time to settle down: the need to establish himself as an individual in a strange new group may lead to over-dominating, or to other forms of exaggerated behaviour. It is relatively easy to make practical preparations for a new arrival: to arrange a written statement of policy and objectives, to arrange a welcoming cup of tea, to allow time to unpack and become familiar with the building. It will be much more complex to help a new arrival into the communal group. I have discussed the residential worker's role in this situation in detail elsewhere (Brearley 1977). Broadly, it will involve providing a warm, secure environment and help for the individual to make approaches to the existing group. He may, perhaps, be introduced to one individual resident or member of staff who can take him around the home. The PSSC report suggests that he should be introduced to all the other residents, otherwise he may be too shy to make his own contacts. This will, of course, depend on the structure of the home and the style of the residential worker. Most importantly a new arrival should not be abandoned in a sitting room full of strangers without being given a way into conversation.

Before an old person is admitted the head of the home

should have received information about him from the field worker. The details which a social worker collects are specialized and gathered for a particular purpose. It is not essential to the decision on whether admission is necessary to know whether an old lady has always had pie and chips on Thursday evenings and chocolate pudding on Sunday but such details can be very important to her contentment in the home. The settling-in period is a process of discovery of the resident's likes and dislikes, and of the home's demands in return. Once a relationship of mutual trust and respect develops the resident can relax and begin to be himself.

Various time limits have been given to the settling-in period. Tobin and Lieberman suggest that when the older person actually enters the home he enters a period of acute disequilibrium for one or two months but after two months the picture is much like that before admission. The first month or two are often described as a period of change and disturbance and it must be recognized that old people will continue to change after admission. Their needs do not necessarily remain the same simply because they are in residential care. It is therefore important to consider their situation after admission and to review their needs. A review three months after admission is important and thereafter a regular, though not necessarily frequent, review should be held.

Continuing contact with the field worker is also desirable. With some clients this may simply be one visit to tidy up loose ends but with others it may involve several visits over a period of months to help the old person to adjust. It has been shown that feelings of separation and abandonment are important elements in poor adjustment and the social worker can help to offset these feelings. He should certainly not add to them by abandoning the old person and emphasizing the feelings of rejection.

THE GERIATRIC TEAM

The problems experienced by old people are rarely simple. They usually involve a combination of factors, breakdown commonly resulting from what Saul (1974) has called the cluster of circumstances. To work effectively with the elderly therefore requires the involvement of a variety of health care and social service professionals. The provision of residential care is very much on the borderline of health and social services. It has even been argued (Lowther and McCleod 1974) that if homes are going to be used to house large numbers of elderly and disabled people then staffing and facilities should become the joint concern of social work and health authorities. Although the DHSS (1977) memorandum of guidance for health care arrangements in homes makes it clear that the care to be provided should be equivalent to that provided by relatives there can be no doubt that residential care involves assessment of a wide range of factors. In so far as they provide new and different relationships for old people all members of the geriatric team contribute to important life changes. The social worker does not have a monopoly of social change and each member of the geriatric team should be aware of the impact of his interaction on the elderly client's or patient's functioning (Brearley 1978).

Admission to care therefore requires the coordinated skills of doctors and nurses as well as field social workers and residential workers. A full assessment of need should include the medical perspective as well as the social perspective. Lowther and McCleod (1974) found that 36 per cent of people admitted to residential care should have been admitted to hospital rather than to a home; a further 39 per cent although considered disabled would have merited a full geriatric assessment. Residential resources are scarce and the demand is considerable; it seems at the very least wasteful to use these resources without careful assessment.

In hazardous situations, when risks are being taken and borne the best protection for all professionals lies in good standards of practice. If there is full assessment and discussion and a team decision is made then it seems more likely that all the relevant considerations will be examined. The client and the workers will be *assured* of a good service and at the same time the workers will be *insured* in so far as they will be free from blame if loss or damage results from the decision. This will apply, of course, only if discussion has been careful and complete and it is important not to use case conferences or team meetings for 'passing the buck'. A team decision should be clearly stated and written down.

One final point should be repeated. In discussing the team it is easy to forget the key figure – the old person, and his family. No decision should be imposed except, perhaps, in the case of advanced brain failure.

SUMMARY

There is a difference between ageing as a process, and old age as a chronologically defined time of life. We are all involved in growing old, and ageing is not a problem, but as individuals proceed through life they may encounter problems. There are some situations which characterize the later part of life, such as retirement, and widowhood, but most people cope with any problems associated with these events with the help of family and friends. It is only a minority who find problems with which they cannot deal without the help of professionals. Some of the general hazards of old age have been outlined: very old age, low income, poor housing, etc. Specific hazards such as ill-health, brain failure, malnutrition, and hypothermia have also been discussed. Residential resources at the present time are in considerable demand and those who are admitted have generally been exposed to an extreme combination of hazards and would be in great danger if they remained in the community.

Old people being admitted to care are therefore in poor physical health and sometimes poor mental health and have been subject to social and emotional stress. The process of admission – of moving from one environment to another – is stressful and, research has shown, can be associated with deterioration and death. It is therefore essential that very vulnerable old people are only exposed to the additional hazard of admission following a careful consideration of whether the potential gains outweigh the potential losses: admission is a risk-taking activity for social workers and clients.

The effects of the admission process can be offset by careful preparation and efficient transfer procedures, involving the old person in discussion and clarification at all stages. Whether or not there is a negative outcome depends also on the quality of the institutional environment. The field worker, residential worker, and other members of the geriatric team must therefore work together to ease the old person through the hazards and dangers of entry to the new environment. That environment should provide physical care and the opportunity for the old person to continue to grow and change within the residential group.

A final, cautionary note must be added. In a paper on relocation research and policy and practice Morton Lieberman (1974) has pointed out that discussion and preparation for the period of transition is an important contribution to preventing unhappiness and feelings of loss. He adds, however, that it may play a relatively small part in reducing the risk because transition to institutional care involves the individual in radical changes and the people admitted to care are ill-equipped for the relearning necessary. We should remember, in other words, that many of the people being admitted are very frail and dependent – the least likely to adapt and perhaps the least likely to survive. Social workers can expect to ease the distress of admission but, in terms of current policy, admission to care remains a risky experience for old people.

8 The Decision to Admit: Policy Framework and Practice

Glenys Jones

As the introduction to the second half of this book has in- dicated, the three preceding chapters have been concerned with two particular themes: the importance of the decision to admit, and the importance of the process of admission. This chapter is primarily concerned with the former. The focus of discussion is on the range of services provided by Social Services Depart- ments (in the context of the whole framework of services provided by health and social services agencies) in terms of how this range can be used to present alternatives to admission to care. While the focus is, therefore, less on the process of admission and rather on the decision to admit the questions raised may nevertheless have an important effect on the process.

It is important to recognize that there is a difference between the range of services provided – the overall development and deployment of resources – and the use of those resources by social worker and client in an operational situation. This might be seen as the difference between social policy, and social work – both of which have a contribution to make to this discussion. It is clear that the risks involved at the policy and planning levels are different from those at the service delivery point. Risks to the agency and community for instance, occur when there is an imbalance between the range of services, where the lack of domiciliary services creates undue pressure on the residential resources. The main questions with which managers, planners, and politicians are concerned are those involving the strategic balancing of services, and hazards arise in the attempt to meet need within the constraints of finance, time, capital developments, and staffing. At a tactical level, on the other hand, risks are involved in the choices the social worker makes in his day-to-day work with clients. Danger may arise in consequence, for instance, of faulty judgement if a decision is taken without adequate information.

The main theme of this chapter, then, is a consideration of the relationship between these two perspectives – the broader policy issues, and the operation of service delivery – and of their implications for the decision to admit, or not to admit to residential care. In order to simplify the discussion it has been decided to use the example of services for the elderly to highlight the main issues.

POLICY FRAMEWORKS

In taking an overview of the services provided for a client group there are several ideas that can be discussed in an attempt to envisage the strategic framework within which services have been developed. These will be briefly examined with their implications for residential care and the nature of the risks associated with them.

(1) Continuum of Care

This idea assumes an increasing severity of individual need. For example, in looking at the elderly, old age would be viewed as a process of increasing mental and physical deterioration over a period of time. As needs increase so different services are provided to match the increasing dependence of the individual. An elderly person, therefore, might require in sequence, befriending services, domiciliary services, sheltered housing, residential care, and finally hospitalization. This implies that each service has a clear boundary, and contains a monitoring and assessment process. The concept of a continuum has implications for the development of a range of services to meet the various degrees of need. The assessment and monitoring functions implied by this model are primarily part of the tactical approach utilized by the social worker in matching the individual client to the service progression.

Whereas the overall strategy must be concerned with the whole range of services on the continuum, it is not necessary for the tactical decision to involve a movement throughout this range. Services are used as a way of achieving efficiency and minimizing professional and client risk bearing. Admission to residential care is seen as an appropriate step in the process of growing individual dependence. After a careful assessment of the client's needs a residential placement is considered to be necessary and the dangers the client may face if not correctly placed, and the hazards to the agency of incorrectly placing the client are assumed to be reduced. The idea of a continuum of care may, however, be based on the false assumption that clients will perceive their own increasing needs and will be willing to undergo the constant changes implied in meeting these needs, to the extent of foregoing the satisfactions of a permanent relationship and the security of a familiar environment. If clients are, in fact, unwilling to be exposed to constant change then it is likely that this model primarily minimizes risks to the agency who provide the range of services, but increases risks to the client who may refuse to use this progression.

(2) Substitution

A related argument is based on the assumption that different services can be used to meet similar needs. This argument is also closely related to the suggestion that older people should be able to choose the kind of service they would like. In the context of the idea of a continuum of care it is probably most likely that the worker will be in a position of choice in so far as he is able to choose from a range of different possibilities to provide the 'right' service for the older person.

In order to create choice for the older person it is necessary to offer at least two services, each of which will offer a comparable level of care. The choice will then be between, for example, being well looked after at home, with a high level of domiciliary resources, voluntary care, support from neighbours, etc., or being well looked after in an old people's home. Alternatively there may be a choice for the older person of taking a place in one of two or three similar old people's homes. Only if services provide an equivalent quality or quantity of service can they be regarded as substitutable and only then can choice be regarded as a reality.

Implicit, also, in the idea of substitution is an assumption about the basic similarity of needs – that very different approaches to meeting needs can be used with similar effect. It is, however, arguable whether 'good care' in a residential institution (however good the regime and environment) can ever be as attractive to most people as 'good care' in their own, familiar home. In other words substitution may tend to be reductionist in effect as it may minimize the differences between people and between the subjective, experiential elements of apparently similar needs. One difficulty of substitutability as a model for planning is that choice is dictated by subjective criteria of need: in practice the decision may be based on the expedience of a course of action rather than on its acceptability to the individual.

(3) Network

The concept of a network of services is based on a system of joint rational planning by a number of disciplines and departments. A clear understanding of the numbers and needs of client groups, it is argued, results in a rational network of services. Clients move appropriately in and out, and across services as their needs occur. With the introduction into local government of ideas of corporate planning in 1972 (see, for example, Bains Committee Report 1972) and the reorganization of 1974 this logical planning of services seemed an achievable objective. In particular research projects have attempted to establish such networks in, for example, services for the elderly in Wessex (Kushlik and Blunden 1974) and for the mentally handicapped in Sheffield (Evaluation Research Group, University of Sheffield 1977). A service network is created in an attempt to accurately and rationally meet client need. This implies a heavy financial commitment and, because of this financial and political accountability, the network tends to be a publicly controlled development. This may underestimate the contribution of alternative provisions in the voluntary and private sectors. A network system may also lead to an inherent conservatism in services as the high cost increases the element of public risk. A partnership with the voluntary sector might result in more risks being taken with more radical experiments that would fit uneasily and with difficulty into an established statutory network.

The service network would include residential care as part of a range of services. Clients would be allocated to different services as considered appropriate to their needs. This form of rationalization might minimize the hazards to the individual agency through collective planning, but for the client the dangers of 'slipping through the net' increase as the need for inter-agency cooperation increases. This model can extend and incorporate the notions of the continuum of care, and of substitution in that it recognizes the desirability of having a range of services providing options – some of which will be very different and some of which will be similar to each other.

(4) Responsive Models of Service

Here the development of services is seen as reactive and is in response to developments in other areas of policy. For Social Service Departments this may imply that services will be provided for 'social casualties' and that this agency will provide a 'fail-safe' device for the limitations of policies or services in other areas. To an extent this role can be seen in an historical perspective of welfare services. The social casualty role can be clearly seen in the 1948 National Assistance Act, while the fail-safe mechanism can be seen in the evolution of policies of community care. The 1959 Mental Health Act and the 1962 Hospital Plan both proposed a higher turnover of patients who would be discharged more quickly into the community. Local authorities were to respond to this by developing and expanding services for prevention and care in the community. For a variety of reasons there was a lack of congruence between practice in the health service and provision in the social services (for a fuller discussion see Roberts (1976)). In the field of care of the elderly during this period residential staff were under increasing pressure with the changing composition of the resident group in old people's homes. It could be argued that a responsive role has importance in providing flexibility to enable other services to take innovative risks. In this framework the Social Service Department provides services for the most disadvantaged members of society and those for whom other agencies cannot, or can no longer provide. Residential care in these terms is likely to provide a mixed population of clients with a wide and disparate range of conditions. Those not clearly falling into the ambit of another agency, yet exhibiting high need, are likely to fall back on the residential sector. Other agencies can limit their risk through rules excluding certain groups but Social Services, by having no such boundaries, and by acting as a last resort, have to accept responsibility for a clientèle who may have a large variety of extensive needs. The danger to the clients may be small in that they have the assurance that this agency has an ultimate responsibility to help.

(5) Welfare Promotion

It is sometimes implied that the agency can make a contribution to major developments in social life: that positive developments can be initiated in a field that is the unique responsibility of that agency. Again, historically it is possible to see the Seebohm Report as attempting to move Social Service Departments from a responsive framework to an innovative one. The stretching and redefining of agency boundaries from responsibility for social casualties to the responsibility for community development is part of this innovative move. Similarly Townsend's insistence on the need for Social Service Departments to have a promotional programme concerned with the equalization of resources, the reduction of isolation, the value of family support and community integration can be seen as an attempt to reinforce this orientation (Townsend 1970). In this framework the agency would be primarily concerned with the promotion of altruism, preventive strategies, and social education across a wide spectrum. Educative and proselytizing functions would be the dominant approaches seeking to create a community. Residential care within this framework would involve innovative approaches including experimenting with a variety of group living situations such as mixed age and ability communes, extensive boarding out schemes, intensive rehabilitation and assessment programmes. Within an innovative framework risks to the agency and client are high because uncertainty is high due to the experimental implication of innovation. Innovation may be restricted to a research project with close monitoring in an attempt to minimize the effects of uncertainty. However, within this framework the ends are sometimes considered to justify the means.

TABLE 8(1) *Summary of frameworks*

framework	description	residential care	risks
continuum of care	range of services to cater for increasingly high needs	as part of chain of services, a penultimate stepping stone to hospital	to agency, low to client, high
substitution	range of services to be used for similar needs	as one of a range of services in a situation of free choice	to agency, high to client, high
network	wide range of interrelated services	as part of service network	to agency, low to client, high
responsive	services adapt to needs thrown up by other agencies	as last resort	to agency, high to client, low
welfare promotion	services seek to promote social well-being	as an experimental living situation	to agency, high to client, low

Social workers may consider that a generalized consideration of frameworks, as attempted above, is an idealistic exercise. However, without such an overall consideration the aims and objectives of agency policy may remain negative and confused. This can result in poor or inappropriate services. Furthermore without such a consideration social workers may constantly feel pressurized while dealing with crises not of their making and outside their control. This in turn can lead to a divergence between ideas they hold about their job and the actual practice of that job. It is important for the development of social work services that questions about the boundaries or potential of welfare services are made more explicit. This is particularly so given the suggestion already made earlier in this book that social workers are dealing with the balancing of uncertainties with the attendant risks that this implies. Until the wider implications and social assumptions concerning the role of welfare services are debated the nature of the risks and responsibilities of social workers, managers, policy makers, and politicians will remain unclear.

Within the consideration of this broader framework one perspective does, however, become clearer. In one sense it is possible to consider 'alternatives to residential care' in terms of the range of provision. This may be in terms of a continuum, or a network of alternatives which may be options in that they provide equivalent levels of service or in that they offer different possibilities to meet different needs. In the day-to-day context of social work with older people, the focus is likely to be on the decision to use one resource or service rather than another. Local and individual variations in provision, combined with issues of felt need in the individual situation are likely to be at least as important to the social worker and his client as are the general perspectives so far discussed.

SERVICES AS ALTERNATIVES

There are considerable difficulties in attempting a categorization of services within the Social Services Department and the division which follows is, of course, somewhat arbitrary. The division has been made to clarify the exploration of the nature of the resources which are available *in addition to* residential care. It is recognized that residential care has been, and continues to be a major area of provision but such care is only one of several alternatives (bearing in mind the cautionary notes which have already been introduced about the concepts of 'alternatives', 'options', and 'suitability'). Residential care need not be a last resort for the older person, either in the sense that there is no other form of service, or in the sense that it is the last place in which the old person lives before death. It can be a positive part of the total range of service to older people: the decision to admit is not necessarily a decision made in despair.

A. Personal Services in Social Services Departments

A sample of such services may include those outlined in *Table 8(2).*

TABLE 8(2)

service	objective
1 *Casework techniques* (including counselling, life review, interpersonal communications, family therapy, modified behaviour modelling, etc)	Relieves anguish. Helps to resolve individual or family tensions. Leads to a feeling of self worth and can lead to better functioning and more appropriate behaviour. *Danger* − without careful input and planning this service can lead to a possible increase in feelings of depression and chance of suicidal feelings.
2 *Advice services*	Accurate information. Improves basic fabric of life and widens areas of choice. *Danger* − without back-up of advocacy this may lead to frustration, withdrawal, continuing need, and risk.

TABLE 8(2)—cont.

service	objective
3 *Befriending services*	These limit social isolation for housebound. This widens the social network and increases feelings of security, companionship, role satisfaction, and selfworth. *Danger* – without careful selection, supervision, or support this service could lead to an inappropriate relationship with the chance of exploitation, rejection, or disillusion.
4 *Domiciliary services* (e.g. Home Help service)	Keep house clean. Decrease social isolation. Provide additional home-making services. This leads to increased confidence in surroundings and better self esteem. *Danger* – without careful assessment this service could lead to inappropriate service and the chance of injury.
5 *Individual protection schemes*	This leads to increased feeling of security, and confidence in the environment. May decrease social isolation. *Danger* – without continuous assessment this service could lead to a sense of false security, by agency and client, and carries the chance of e.g. undetected fall.

Discussion

A wide range of personal services can be offered to the elderly. It is usually accepted that these services should be available to anyone who needs them, although it is recognized that in practice not everyone in need is actually referred for help. The comments on these services apply across the range of Social Service Department client groups. While the strengths of each particular service can be indicated, it should be noted that each service tends to have a dual function affecting personal and social wellbeing. The balance between these two tends to have a different emphasis in different services, e.g. the range of counselling techniques are primarily concerned with intrapersonal or interpersonal wellbeing; however, when inner tensions and stress are relieved so better social functioning often occurs. Similarly the practical tasks of the Home Help may encourage feelings of wellbeing in an improved environment, while also reducing feelings of loneliness and sense of loss through companionship and practical support. Each personal service although having these dual functions needs a particular input of skill or knowledge. It is important, therefore, to clarify the role boundaries within the various services. Particular skills and knowledge are needed to provide, for example, Advice and Advocacy services, and these may be different from those needed to provide counselling help. Despite this awareness of role difference, however, human need is not as clearly differentiated. Consequently within the agency, regular supervision, teamwork, and planning are necessary to maintain awareness of the inter-relationship of human needs. There are two main ways in which the agency can minimize risk to itself in the provision of personal services. One is by ensuring that its staff have the skills, knowledge, and controls necessary to their prime function, and the second is by the reinforcement of the agency's commitment to attempts to meet individual human needs. These points both imply a clear understanding of agency and professional responsibility and reinforce the value of training for agency staff. Professional control is also implied with the emphasis on the sharing of information, and the necessity of supervision and careful teamwork. Among the main hazards to the client are an unknowledgeable helper and an uncaring agency.

In the range of personal services outlined above hazards occur at several points. First, when the services mentioned are not provided at all and no alternative ways of meeting needs emerge. Consequently an elderly, isolated person is in danger of not receiving any service. Second, hazards arise when the services are provided but are inadequate either because of lack of knowledge and skill, lack of consistency and reliability, or lack of resources leading to incomplete or inadequate services. Third, there are difficulties when services are provided but are inappropriate and consequently fail to meet individual levels of need in any particular circumstances. The dangers attached to these conditions will be examined briefly.

The dangers attendant upon not providing services when there is a moral and social responsibility to do so are such that individual suffering increases, agency risk increases, and there may be a decline in social awareness and caring in the community. Services that are offered and refused present a different problem to those that arise when services are not offered when a need is apparent. As so many responsibilities in the development of services for the elderly reside in permissive powers the issue of providing services to meet needs is an area of concern for agencies. It is difficult for them to measure needs: one measure of need lies in the nature of referral to the agency but it is important to take account of other forms of need. In identifying such other needs there are several strategies that agencies can pursue including wider publicity; diversifying resources to key agencies, e.g. GPs' hospitals, volunteer bureaux, churches etc.; the introduction of review registers; or encouraging forms of community work. Broadening the base of agency responsibilities can reduce hazards and minimize danger.

When services are provided but for a variety of reasons are inadequate, agencies may feel satisfied that they are providing *something*, yet, in fact, the risk to the agency may be greater as contact in itself implies social responsibilities. To the client the hazards attendant upon raising hopes, providing a false consciousness of security and activity but without adequately meeting needs may result in heightened feelings of helplessness, frustration, and depression. The danger is that this could result in abuse, withdrawal, hypothermia, suicide, or even a painful and premature death. Whilst risk is clearly seen in child abuse cases, with the elderly the 'mask' of self-determination can hide service weakness.

The inadequacy of personal services can be indicated by two examples. First in the casework field. As previously mentioned there has been a degree of disinterest, and sometimes reluctance on the part of skilled personnel to use their skills for the elderly. The reorganizations that in particular have affected hospital social work have possibly led to a decrease in this service in the health sector, whilst work attachment to general practice is not a widespread phenomenon. The skills involved in bereavement counselling for example, have been developed by volunteer groups (Age Concern 1977b), rather than by Social Service Department staff. Similarly the interpersonal skills involved in counselling work in the individual, marital, or family fields have rarely been offered to elderly clients. Whilst the need for these skills may be relatively small it is nevertheless apparent (Goldberg, Mortimer, and Williams 1970). Second, domiciliary services are often provided in a limited or inadequate form. A recent study in London stated that 'Many old people in need of care and support, and supposedly "receiving domiciliary services", are living in miserable and distressing physical conditions' (Plank 1977). Social workers are increasingly aware of the limitations of these services in the form in which they are provided (Jones 1978). As there are more older people with increasingly high needs living in the community, so the demand for more intensive domiciliary services grows. This ranges through the need for incontinence services, nightsitting services, seven-day meal services, and home helps in the form of family aids or daily home-making services. The more intensive use of domiciliary services can have repercussions for other services. For example, volunteer befriending schemes may be used to supplement the home help service. Volunteers may be used to take on some of the tasks previously performed by home helps, such as shopping, washing, etc. The inter-relationship and appropriateness of the personal services, therefore, needs careful and imaginative planning.

When services are provided but considered by the client or agency to be inappropriate, this may be the result of inadequate assessment, inadequacy of resources, misplacement, or a reflection of the severity of a person's condition or situation. Inappropriate service delivery may also occur when – as often happens – both health and social services workers are involved with an old person. A multidisciplinary approach to assessment and service delivery is necessary to ensure appropriate and adequate services are provided.

Another issue that arises when considering the personal services is the question of who should provide the service. In a pluralist society many of the tasks described above are performed by a variety of agencies, not only statutory agencies but churches, advice bureaux, voluntary agencies, and agencies covering both the public and private sector, and those involving both professionals and volunteers. This pluralism has implications for the role of Social Service Departments. Hadley, Webb, and Farrell (1975:192) argue that Social Service Departments could be the public body assigned overall responsibilities for providing services for the isolated and lonely. They echo the belief held by many that: 'It is only through the local authority that a comprehensive, regular and reliable service to old people will be provided.' Whilst some local authorities may not wish to accept such wide-ranging responsibilities the main task of the authority could well of that of delegation, coordination, partnership, and supervision of private and voluntary agencies and volunteer groups. This would increase the involvement of the Social Service Department in promotional, educative, and community support activities. This in turn may lead to a more accurate, high-need referral for intensive service delivery that could minimize the hazards attendant upon the inappropriate or inadequate delivery of services.

In themselves the personal social services have much to offer that can affect the quality of life of individuals. In so far as these services can be considered as alternatives to residential care, however, it can be seen that by themselves they are extremely limited. Personal services may be used intensively as a temporary measure prior to admission. When this is the case the risk to the client and the agency is high in the sense that danger is both imminent and serious although it may be that the services provide an essential 'holding' operation. Here the risk of *not* admitting directly must be borne.

It is possible that the range of personal services can be used to provide true alternatives for the individual, through the use of services in combination. The development of integrated home care programmes by Social Service Departments, and schemes such as Hospital at Home developed by the National Health Service reveal the potential of combination (Association of County Councils 1979; Lang 1976). The most intensive form of personal service in the community remains fostering and this is likely to be limited with the elderly and elderly mentally infirm. Where it does occur it is usually described as 'boarding-out', or 'lodgings' and has particular potential as a short-stay alternative. The fact that the givers of this service are themselves often elderly also indicates that for this alternative to be more widespread a similar range of supportive services will be necessary for the care givers themselves.

The use of personal services as alternatives to residential care poses different problems for Social Service Departments dependent upon whether the elderly person lives alone, with family, or with a substitute family. The role of the social worker would change, as Plank (1979) has suggested, and they might become 'case managers' who would coordinate and mobilize support services. Similarly the task of agency management would change, particularly at the area level. Here the coordination and stimulation of a variety of local initiatives would be given priority. The professional task for the Social Service Department would be to act as a 'knowledge bank' to promote and feed good ideas to voluntary groups and to act as supervisors for ongoing voluntary schemes. Limited financial support but with the support of professional expertise could result in a wider preventive and socially supportive network for many vulnerable groups.

For social services to aim to provide an alternative by offering intensive delivery to high-need cases, could have the effect of reducing services to the low-need client groups. At present we do not know how far the delivery of minimum services to the elderly and their families acts as a preventive measure. To withdraw such service without substituting other social supports could be premature and lead to an actual increase in the number of vulnerable old people in need in the community.

B. Group Support Services in Social Service Departments

A sample of such services may include Social Clubs and Day Care.

TABLE 8(3)

service	objective
1 *Social Clubs*	Provides companionship, widens the range of activities and interests of members. Could increase mobility and self esteem and social skills of members. *Danger* – can lead to complacency if used primarily by those already with social contacts. Clique formation can isolate others. Reliance on transport system for housebound.
2 *Day Care*	Provides companionship. Widens the range of contacts for elderly person. Provides food and warmth. Can relieve family pressure. *Danger* – can lead to complacency if no adequate programme provided. May heighten vulnerability at night time or weekend. Reliance on transport system for housebound.

Discussion

The forms of care outlined in *Table 8(3)* require older people to leave their homes for a period of time and these services are, therefore, reliant on ease of access and transport. The characteristic of this form of care is that it provides various kinds of peer group activity with the mutual support and self help this may involve. The main advantages of this form of service is that it provides an out-of-home focus for people who may have no other alternative social focus. It may provide a lively, enjoyable contact that widens the scope of individual interests, and provides a meeting place for others, so that the elderly person may have some choice in the selection of friends.

When these forms of group activities are organized and managed on a democratic basis it may also reawaken or introduce the recipient to new roles and responsibilities, and hence widen the person's ability to control their own environment.

It is arguable how far Social Service Departments should be involved in providing such facilities. On the one hand social clubs and centres have been seen to be the particular focus of the voluntary sector, with on the other hand, day care more properly the focus of the statutory sector. It may, however, be useful to highlight the areas of similarity between the two. Both forms of activity involve, at least to some extent, relieving social isolation by bringing people together. The main skills utilized by professionals within these activities are those of group work, and organizational and interpersonal skills.

If we consider social clubs it is true that a wide variety of groups exist in the community, many of which are supported by older people and are positively encouraged by Social Service Departments. Many such groups are limited in that they have a particular bias which is generally accepted by the membership, e.g. church-based social clubs. The argument for a Social Service Department's duplicating these lies in the wider concern of this Department with the wellbeing of the person who may be considered unacceptable within these established groups or clubs. Amongst the elderly the reclusive, the mentally deteriorating, the addicted, the isolated, and the immobile person may be introduced to a social group as part of a long-term commitment to support or rehabilitation.

One possible limitation of group support services is that they involve age segregation. The dangers associated with such social group involvement can, therefore, paradoxically include that of increased social withdrawal into a peer or problem group. It may also lead to isolation within the peer group so that the increasingly deaf, immobile, or mentally deteriorating member may be excluded from functions which become the prerogative of an active clique. A further danger is that of increased boredom when there is a repetitious or limited range of activities, e.g. the bingo phenomenon. The problems of boredom, clique formation, age segregation, and the withdrawal of individual members were all successfully tackled by a British study of Northcote House Senior Club, where a self education and activities programme was established. This led those conducting the study to conclude that 'the role of staff in hospitals, day centres and clubs is to keep the elderly totally in touch with reality and the world around them, harsh as that world may be rather than enfolding them in a too protective atmosphere which begins insidiously to isolate them from the community' (Lewis and Oldfield 1977).

Given these brief comments consideration will now be given to how far group support services may contribute to offsetting the need for admission to residential care. Increasingly it is being suggested that the potential in these services lies in two areas. The first is in the area of prevention. A premise behind the Northcote House Senior Club was that 'Such services should seek to prevent the crises which lead to elderly people having prematurely to be taken into care, or having to be totally supported by the statutory services within their own homes' (Lewis and Oldfield 1977:5). Similarly Post (1965:76) suggests that 'lack of social contacts and of opportunities to keep up interests and skills may hasten or even precipitate senile dementia'. The second area of potential lies in the introduction of the elderly to a social group following a crisis: these services can act as part of a rehabilitation programme. Discharge for an elderly hospital patient might include attendance at a day hospital followed by transfer to a Social Service Department day centre and attendance at out-patient clinic. Pitt (1974:107) suggests that this pattern 'offers a real alternative to admission, promotes discharges and offers continuing support to many patients who would otherwise relapse and have to be readmitted again and again'. Successful group care depends upon appropriate referrals, access and transportation, and a thoughtful social programme.

Given this potential the role of Social Service Departments with respect to the development of group services needs to be carefully considered. Group services can do much to improve the quality of life of individual elderly persons and there are many small groups already in existence in the community.

Through voluntary liaison committees, small grants, and educative support Social Service Departments can do much to stimulate and encourage these groups. Support may often be necessary to enable groups to expand their activities or lower their level of tolerance and be more accepting of disadvantaged members. With encouragement groups can also expand their activities to make links with members who are housebound at time of crises. Social Service Departments could perform a useful promotional role in this area. By providing their own day centres they could also offer a more intensive form of social provision to the more handicapped elderly person in the community. This could then be seen as a reliable and continuous preventive or rehabilitative device. The potential of such group care services depends upon a careful appraisal of the aims and objectives of each group and it is therefore important to recognize the need for group skills, incorporating rehabilitative aims. Such a focus could also lead to a greater development of group work in the residential setting. Day care or regular contact with a social group may be seen as a way of both the agency and client minimizing hazards but the most disabled client will continue to be exposed to hazards in the evenings or weekends. To provide a service equivalent to that which is currently available in the residential situation, therefore, these services would need to function in combination with other services.

C. Total Care Services in Social Service Departments

The main example from Social Service Departments is Residential care.

TABLE 8(4)

service	objective
Residential care	To provide for those 'in need of care and attention which is not otherwise available to them'. A characteristic of this care is that it provides 24 hour, 7 day a week cover in a segregated environment.

TABLE 8(4)—cont.

service	objective
	Danger − any move of an elderly person from a familiar environment to a strange one increases the likelihood of death. The effects of institutionalization can introduce the possibility of social, physical, and mental atrophy.

Discussion

Residential care provided by Social Service Departments has a number of features in common with other forms of accommodation provided by other agencies, such as sheltered housing and hospital care. An objective of this care is to provide an environment in which the whole person can thrive. Unfortunately this objective is often subsumed under other tasks which the agency may consider important, such as the overall appearance of the unit, the importance of time keeping and routine, the safety of the individual, etc. Whilst these tasks may serve to reduce hazards, when they become dominant they are in danger of reducing the humanity of both staff and residents. A further weakness of this sector is that it is often staffed by untrained or partially trained personnel who may be working with clients suffering from a sense of personal trauma, loss of identity, and with high dependancy needs. This combination of staff and client weakness can be very hazardous. The older person in residential care may be confronted by a series of personal crises such as the loss of significant others, the loss of a faculty, or approaching death, and is therefore likely to be in need of sensitive and careful understanding and personal help and guidance. The staff themselves may be in the position of needing guidance, supervision, and support in coping with these situations. Admission to total care carries its own risks but these are likely to be greater for the client than for the staff. For the client the loss of personal identity and self esteem and the trauma of entry to total care can lead to depression, aggression, or death. The staff are exposed to the dangers of depression and withdrawal, and becoming defensive and insensitive to the needs of residents.

There is an ambiguity within Social Service Departments concerning the appropriate purpose of residential care for the elderly. It may be helpful at this stage to briefly review the development of residential care for the elderly before examining its potential development. The origins of local authority old people's homes lie in the political reconstructions following World War Two. The intention in 1948 was to abolish the local authority workhouse and provide small, community-based hostels for the elderly. Here it was intended that they could maintain their independence whilst their personal needs were catered for. Old people's homes were to provide a form of protective social living for those who chose this (see Hansard 1948). The idea of a state-provided hotel was supported. This analogy with a hotel contained the idea of greater equality between the classes, of providing a dignified, humane, and destigmatized living arrangement for the elderly, and presented a viable alternative to the workhouse. The historical focus, therefore, was on the clientèle who needed care but who were not able to get it in any other form. This allowed room for the development of alternative services.

With the continued expansion of domiciliary services since 1963 it has been suggested that 'the more these can be expanded the more pressure on residential accommodation and on hospitals can be eased' (DHSS 1976d:41). One argument then, is based on the assumption that if more alternative services could be provided then the need for residential care will decline. That this has not occurred is partly because developments in related health care sectors have counterbalanced this effect. It might also be that the demand on old people's homes to admit increasingly infirm and totally dependent residents is a reflection of the success of alternative services. The more services are used to provide support for older people previously admitted to care the more the residential sector will be dealing with the heavily dependent, and the overlap between this sector and the hospital services will increase. Local authority old people's homes have increasingly been admitting very infirm residents so that 'staff in old people's homes are coming under increasing pressure due to the rapid increase in the numbers of residents who would previously have been admitted to geriatric wards'.* This despite the fact that 'the staff of a home are not expected to provide a professional kind of health care that is properly the function of the primary health care services. Nor should residential homes be used as nursing homes or extensions of hospitals' (DHSS/Welsh Office 1977). However, the considerable dependency needs of residents, and the limitations of the domiciliary services already mentioned have meant that old people's homes have occupied an intermediate position between the hospital and community support systems. Residential care for the elderly balances uneasily between these two.

The Personal Social Services Council suggest that residential care should provide for one or more of the following − 'assessment and re-assessment, day care, education and training, holiday relief for client or his family, maintenance of client's condition, protection, refuge, rehabilitation, social training, terminal care, therapy' (PSSC 1977 : 10). Many of these are not currently provided for the elderly clientèle of Social Services Departments, who may well be able to benefit from them. The use of short-term stays in residential homes for assessment, holiday relief, day care, rehabilitation, and social training could well lead to a reduction in the need for long-stay admission to care. The total care of the most vulnerable, dependent, and impaired older people could become the joint responsibility of the National Health Service and Social Services Departments and many elderly people currently misplaced, or in a hazardous independent − or assisted-independent − situation, could benefit from a more constructive period of short-stay residence. The use of short-stay care − in combination with community support services − could, therefore, act as a viable alternative to long-stay residential care for some people.

CONCLUDING

To return to the initial theme it is clear that the decision to

---

* Editorial report *Social Work Today* **8** (18):3.

admit to care has to be made within a very complex range of constraints and possibilities. At a general level policy-makers and planners are concerned with the obvious fact that different people have different needs and it is therefore necessary to create a variety of different services to accommodate to individual situations. On an operational level social workers, and others involved in the delivery of services to older people, are concerned to put together collections of coordinated services for individuals.

In examining the decision to admit the idea of 'alternatives to residential care' has been used. This is a difficult concept which appears to have a number of meanings and by way of clarification some summary points can be made.

(1) Residential care provides, for the elderly, a level of personal care which is rarely available in the community because of the limited amount of domiciliary provision which has to be spread thinly among a large (and increasing) number of people. In a theoretical sense it is possible to discuss the creation of a package of services which will provide for the old person, in his own home, the same level of personal care as he would receive in residential care. In practice, however, this remains more of an ideal than a reality and in this sense of an equivalent form of service, alternatives to residential care do not usually exist for older people (Personal Social Services Research Unit 1979).

Similarly the lack of resources affects other age groups and client groups: the lack of suitable foster homes for children may in practice mean that there is 'no alternative' to admission to a Children's Home.

(2) At the same time it should be recognized that residential care may offer positive benefits. Some older people say they wish to enter residential care (although the nature of this desire may be open to debate) and the experience of group living, of warmth, food, and companionship may have the effect of improving the sense of wellbeing and the functioning of some people. The same is again true of children, or of the mentally ill: the institutional environment is not exclusively negative.

Nevertheless there is an overwhelming tendency to regard

residential care as the last resort – in the sense that it is only acceptable if all other possibilities have been explored. In this sense 'alternatives to residential care' can refer simply to other possibilities which may be tried as a way of offsetting, or delaying the need for admission.

(3) It should also be remembered that 'residential care' is a blanket term which itself includes a very wide range of different situations. The provision of alternatives may, therefore, involve giving the client the opportunity to understand the different kinds of residential facility – to visit and explore them if possible – before choosing. There may be a degree of inevitability in the need for residential care in some form but there can still be a measure of individual choice about which home is chosen.

In summary, the careful use of a variety of services can lead to the avoidance of residential care for some older people. Social workers accepted a commitment to explore alternatives to residence in the child-care field in the 1960s,* and more recently in BASW's evidence concerning the review of the Mental Health Act, accepted the same responsibility in relation to the mentally disordered; now such a commitment is needed towards the elderly. The grounds for this commitment lie not in the area of costs, as alternatives may prove to be more expensive than residential care, but on grounds of humanity (see Armitage (1979)). The preference of many people is to live and die in their own homes. This preference carries risks, yet in so far as social work is concerned with individual wellbeing, so this should be a desired objective.

Risk can be minimized by the planning of resources at both the policy and service-delivery levels. The task for the social worker should be to initiate a plan adapted to individual circumstances following a careful assessment of the individual situation. For this to be a feasible objective two conditions have to apply. First, the resources of the social work agency need to be adaptable and extensive. Second, as has happened in cases of

* See discussion of Section 1, Children and Young Persons Act, 1963, in Heywood and Allen (1971).

child abuse, inter-agency cooperative strategies need to be adopted. In particular, the overlapping objectives of the health, personal social services, and housing sectors need to be considered at all levels. Hazards frequently occur for elderly people as, for example, when they are discharged from hospital, or following bereavement, and a joint approach to the problems of the individual can help to minimize the hazards surrounding these incidents. I am, therefore, suggesting that Social Service Departments have a crucial role to play where hazardous situations involving the elderly are concerned. This includes not just reacting to situations as they occur, but seeking to positively identify and develop liaison with GPs, hospitals, and community services.

If alternative strategies are developed then the role of residential care will change. Here the knowledge and insight from social work over the years has much to offer. All staff involved in the long-term total care of the elderly, whatever their discipline or the setting of this care, need an understanding of the social work approach to residential care. As the residential setting becomes the base for a variety of activities such as assessment, day care, and short-term care, it becomes increasingly important that this approach is understood and utilized.

The differential use of residential care, the sharing of this task with other agencies, and the development of intensive alternatives highlight social workers' concern with the client at risk. The proper identification of these clients and the appropriate matching of services to need is likely to remain the dominant concern of the Social Service Department. However, this task in itself involves a wider concern for social wellbeing. Here the task of the agency is to promote, encourage, and support local initiative so that family and neighbourhood concern for the elderly is encouraged.

For the social work agency the residential sector covers a small percentage of clients' needs. In any consideration of risk this percentage is, however, crucial as the traditional approach to reducing this has been by admission to care. Risks may also, however, be minimized by considering a variety of approaches that may reduce the need to admit to residential care, and may also improve the quality of life of the prospective resident. A commitment to the pursuit of alternatives is possible only with the cooperation of other agencies in the statutory and private sectors. Social workers must be skilled in not only analysing the risks in the client situation, but the risks to their own and other agencies. The task of pursuing the wellbeing of the individual is increasingly the result of corporate effort.

Conclusion   *Paul Brearley*

In Chapter 7 attention was drawn to the increasing importance in social work practice of haste, of urgency, and of emergency. The interrelationships of these words with the concepts of risk, vulnerability, and protection, and their careless and haphazard use have important implications for good practice. One principle aim of this book has been to begin a clarification of some of the elements within the use of the term 'risk'. The second major objective of the book has been to explore the nature of admission to care as a process which involves the time and energies of many, if not all social workers and as an experience to which a significant number of people are exposed.

The basic premises can be simply expressed. People are admitted to care because they are vulnerable in their living situation: they are at-risk. However, admission to care is a process which involves its own hazards and similarly living in an enclosed institutional situation involves exposure to particular hazards. It has been argued, therefore, that admission to residential care is not a course of action to be undertaken or advocated lightly. People should ideally enter care only if it is clear that the potential benefits of admission outweigh the potential disadvantages. Unfortunately our ability to predict outcomes is limited by the extent of our knowledge and information, and by chance elements. Particularly important in the context of decision making is the value element. In part values are expressed in the legal, statutory, and organizational frameworks within which social workers operate but individuals will value possible outcomes very differently and a major part of the social work task lies in the clarification of the value components of decision making.

There are two other particularly important themes which have been raised both explicitly and implicitly throughout the book which must be carefully considered. The first of these is choice, and the second is information, with the associated issues of communication.

Choice is often offered as a fundamental right of human beings and it can be argued that it is the ability to choose which distinguishes men and women as rational beings. Yet a discussion of choice is difficult for a number of reasons. In the first place it is not clear what choice means, either as a concept or as a principle for policy or practice. To some extent this difficulty does stem from a confusion between the policy implications of an adherence to the principle of encouraging choice and the practice implications of such a principle. We have already shown, for example, that choice for the elderly has often been presented in terms of the comparability of different forms of care – particularly residential and domiciliary services. But it has also been shown that such care rarely exists: the costs of providing a level of care in the older person's own home equivalent to that available in an old people's home are very great and such comparability does not exist. To talk of choosing between being well looked after at home or being equally well looked after in residential care is unrealistic at present. However there is a difference between creating a set of resources which provides for the fact that different people have different needs and the more individual aspects of choice. Choice exists for the individual when there are at least two options available: there is a difference between choosing which place in a residential home to accept when there are two or three similar places available and choosing between whether to stay at home in very stressful circumstances or to enter residential care and become exposed to a different set of hazards. It should also be repeated here that there is a difference between the choice and the dilemma. There is a choice when at least two options exist and there is a dilemma when there are at least two options each of which is likely to have unpleasant consequences. I recently heard a resident of an old people's home complain that her fellow residents had not taken advantage of the opportunity to choose from a menu: but the options of sago pudding, blancmange, and stewed prunes perhaps hardly offer choice but rather a dilemma! A difficulty of discussing choice, then, is the fact that for many people there may not be a choice between good and less good but between bad and less bad. But, as that resident pointed out, people have a right to know their dilemma.

Although choice has been identified as a right it is, nevertheless, not easy to be clear about why choice is to be valued. Justifications for the important position given to choice are frequently expressed in terms of its contribution to other valued opportunities. In the case of children, for instance, the opportunity to choose can be seen as contributing to learning self reliance, and responsibility. In a recent discussion of services for the elderly a working group of the Personal Social Services Council suggested that 'the aim of all services should be to help people remain as independent as possible and that the starting point for such independence is the availability of a choice of services' (PSSC 1979:9). In this argument the value of choice rests on the value ascribed to independence. However desirable choice may be, the emphasis on it as a desirable feature of life creates a series of dilemmas in the context of admission to care. Questions arise, for instance, about the capacity of a child to make a responsible decision: when should the child be protected from having to make a decision and when should he be given the chance to choose? Similarly it may be asked how social workers are to understand or measure the ability of a mentally disturbed client to make a rational decision. The elderly too may present problems in relation to their ability to decide rationally, or responsibly.

The earlier discussions have also identified the dilemmas which arise when one person's right to choice in a risky situation is likely to expose another to risk. The right of the old person to choose to stay at home may only be made possible at the expense of the health and wellbeing of a neighbour or daughter. Conversely the right of a daughter to choose not to look after her elderly parents may only be exercised at the expense of their health and wellbeing. If we are to assume, therefore, that there is a right to choice then that right must be seen in the context of a corresponding duty to act responsibly towards others.

In order to exercise choice both rationally and responsibly there must be access to information. As Frank Hall points out in Chapter 6 the reality of free choice depends on the existence of alternatives, the person's knowledge of them, and on his freedom from coercion. Knowledge can very rarely be complete and in reality decisions are usually made in the light of limited information. However the social worker can make a substantial contribution to increasing knowledge and available information by improving communication. Lack of information or incorrect information are hazards to the danger of making a wrong decision. If these hazards can be offset by improved communication then a more informed decision can be made.

FIELD WORKER AND RESIDENTIAL WORKER

A further theme that has been raised in later chapters has been the question of communication between field workers and residential workers.

Most people who enter residential care are admitted on the advice of a field social worker. Many people do go into institutions – hospitals, prisons, private and voluntary homes for the elderly, and for the handicapped – without the involvement of social workers, but where social workers are involved it is rare for the residential worker to be the primary worker in the admission process. Often the decision is made with minimal, or even no involvement at all of the residential worker.

A working party report from the Central Council for Education and Training in Social Work (1973:11), in common with many other recent commentators suggests that 'residential work is an intrinsic part of social work, although, like other fields of practice, it has specialised knowledge and skills in addition to the basic elements'. Many of the things that residential workers do involve social work skills and it seems particularly important that a social work service should continue to be available to the new resident. It is essential that field and residential workers should be able to communicate to facilitate the continuing of social work help both during and after admission. Together they are able to offer a more informed service. Cooperation and collaboration are important to facilitate exchange and to ease the admission process: communication is important because it leads to an improved service to clients.

LIVING IN CARE: AFTER ADMISSION

This is not a book about residential care, nor is it intended only to be about field social work but in its concern with that period of transition between an outside environment and residential living it has to consider both field and residential situations.

Four themes have been brought out and have been highlighted in this conclusion. Two themes have been specifically identified and discussed: risk and the process of admission. The second two themes – the importance of choice and responsibility, and of information and communication – have been less explicit but are closely linked to the ideas of good practice which have been expressed throughout. In concluding and summarizing it should be noted that each of these themes also has a relevance to life in residential care.

It has been argued that 'the expectation of society at large and some residents, relatives and staff in particular is that residential care should provide a total, safe risk-free cocoon in which responsibility for all aspects of living is with the provider' (Harris 1977:19). This model of residential care – only one of several – is in some contrast with that which stresses the importance of the resident being able to take risks and responsibility for himself and which was discussed in Chapter 1. The two positions are not necessarily contradictory, although taken to the extreme they may be. It does seem to be important that residential care should provide protection from distress, from exploitation, from physical harm, poverty, etc. Equally it seems important that people in care should be able to explore and face the hazards in their lives and decide for themselves which risks they should take – as long as those risks do not impose unacceptably on others.

The process of admission, to take the second theme, does not end when the door closes behind the new arrival. A question raised in relation to all the groups discussed, and particularly in relation to the mentally ill is when, for the field social worker, does the process end? To dwell on generalizations about time periods for involvement does not seem particularly productive: different people have different needs. The important fact to emphasize is that settling in is a part of a longer process of adjustment: people bring with them needs, interests, and potentials from the past and will continue to grow and change – whatever their age. It is part of the residential worker's task to ensure that the hazards and dangers of institutional living (over-dependence, over-protection, emotional deprivation, lack of stimulation etc.) do not prevent positive development.

Finally, it is important that choice and opportunity in the residential setting are maintained: that people are able, and if necessary are helped, to choose the kind of life they wish to lead within the limits of their environment. They should not only have options available but they should clearly understand what is available and be helped to select where necessary.

FINAL REFLECTIONS

To give proper attention to these questions of residential living requires several more volumes. For the present purposes it should be repeated that admission to care is a very important process and social workers should give very careful attention to working with clients during this process.

As was suggested in the introduction, to admit someone to care is often to be involved in a major life change for an individual and for those around him, usually at a time of distress and crisis. The events that happen during admission to care can be magnified for everyone involved and the things that are done to, with, and around a client at this time often have a lasting effect. What the worker does at such a time is therefore of very great significance.

It must also be emphasized that residential care is not always a last resort: it may be the best solution chosen realistically from a range of alternatives. Residential care should not be seen in purely negative terms: it can and often does offer sanctuary, treatment, security, and real *care*. Social workers must learn to use these positives and possibilities for their clients.

References

Abrams, M. (1978) *Beyond Three Score Years and Ten*. London: Age Concern.

Age Concern (1974) *The Attitudes of the Retired and Elderly*. London: Age Concern.

____ (1975) *Manifesto on the Place of the Retired and the Elderly in Modern Society*. London: Age Concern.

____ (1977a) *Profiles of the Elderly: 3: Aspects of Life Satisfaction*. London: Age Concern.

____ (1977b) Bereavement: Sharing the Pain. *Age Concern Today* **23** (Autumn): 15 – 17.

Anonymous (1978) Consumers Viewpoint: An old folk's home. *Social Work Today* **9** (44): 16.

Armitage, M. (1979) The Cost of Caring for the Elderly. *Social Work Today* **10** (38): 15 – 16.

Association of British Adoption and Fostering Agencies (1977) *Working with Children who are Joining New Families*. London: ABAFA.

____ (undated) *Ending the Waiting. Which Children and What Plan?* London: ABAFA.

____ (1976) *Explaining Adoption: Talking to the Small Child About Adoption*. London: ABAFA.

Association of County Councils (1979) *All Our Future*. London: ACC.

Bacon, R. and Rowe, J. (1978) *Substitute Family Care*: Vol. 1: *The Use and Misuse of Resources*. London: ABAFA.

Bains Committee Report (1972) *The New Local Authorities. Management and Structure*. London: HMSO.

Barnes, G. G. (1978) Communicating with Children. In CCETSW *Study No. 1, Good Enough Parenting*. London: CCETSW.

Barton, R. (1959) *Institutional Neurosis*. Bristol: John Wright.

Bean, P. (1979) The Mental Health Act 1959: Rethinking an Old Problem. *British Journal of Law and Society* **6** (1).

Beedell, C. (1970) *Residential Life with Children*. London: Routledge and Kegan Paul.

Bem, D. J. (1971) The Concept of Risk in the Study of Human Behaviour. In R. E. Carney (ed.) *Risk-Taking Behaviour*. Illinois: Charles C. Thomas.

Berry, J. (1971) Helping Children Directly. *British Journal of Social Work* **1** (3): 315 – 32.

――― (1972a) The Experience of Reception into Residential Care. *British Journal of Social Work* **2** (4): 423 – 34.

――― (1972b) *Social Work with Children.* London: Routledge and Kegan Paul.

Bettelheim, B. (1950) *Love is not Enough.* Ch. 2. New York: The Free Press.

Billis, D. (1973) Entry into Residential Care. *British Journal of Social Work* **3** (4): 447 – 70.

Blascovich, J. and Ginsburg, G. P. (1978) Conceptual Analysis of Risk-Taking in Risky-Shift Research. *Journal for the Theory of Social Behaviour* **8** (2): 217 – 30.

Bloom, M. (1975) *The Paradox of Helping: Introduction to the Philosophy of Scientific Practice.* Chichester: John Wiley.

Bosanquet, N. (1978) *A Future for Old Age.* London: Temple Smith/New Society.

Bowlby, J. (1951) *Maternal Care and Mental Health.* Geneva: World Health Organisation.

――― (1965) *Child Care and the Growth of Love* (2nd edn.). Harmondsworth: Penguin.

――― (1971) *Attachment and Loss* I: *Attachment.* Harmondsworth: Penguin.

――― (1975) *Attachment and Loss* II: *Separation.* Harmondsworth: Penguin.

Bradshaw, J., Emerson, D., and Haxby, D. (1972) Reception to Prison. *British Journal of Social Work* **2** (3): 323 – 35.

Brearley, C. P. (1972) Waiting for Age. *Social Work Today* **3** (18).

――― (1975) *Social Work, Ageing and Society.* London: Routledge and Kegan Paul.

――― (1976a) Social Gerontology and Social Work. *British Journal of Social Work* **6** (4): 433 – 47.

――― (1976b) Old People in Care. *Community Care* (Supplement) October.

――― (1977) *Residential Work with the Elderly.* London: Routledge and Kegan Paul.

――― (1978) Ageing and Social Work. In D. Hobman (ed.) *The Social Challenge of Ageing.* London: Croom Helm.

Brill, K. and Thomas, R. (1964) *Children in Homes.* London: Gollancz.

Brimblecombe, F. S. W. (1976) How About Parents as Partners. *Social Work Service* **9** (April) 19 – 21.

BASW (1975a) Code of Practice: Children at Risk. *Social Work Today* **6** (11).

――― (1975b) *A Code of Ethics for Social Work.* Birmingham: British Association of Social Workers.

_____ (1977a) *Guidelines for Social Work with the Elderly*. Birmingham: British Association of Social Workers.

_____ (1977b) *The Social Work Task*. Birmingham: British Association of Social Workers.

_____ (1977c) *Mental Health Crisis Services – A New Philosophy*. Birmingham: British Association of Social Workers.

Britton, C. (1955) Casework Techniques in the Child Care Services. *Social Casework* **36** (1): January.

Brocklehurst, J. C., Carty, M. H., Leeming, J. T., and Robinson, J. M. (1978) Medical Screening of Old People Accepted for Residential Care. *Lancet*: No. 8081: July 15th.

Brocklehurst, J. (1978) Ageing and Health. In D. Hobman (ed.) *The Social Challenge of Ageing*. London: Croom Helm.

Cang, S. (1976) Why Not a Hospital at Home Then? *Age Concern Today* **20**: 9 – 11.

CCETSW (1973) *Residential Work is part of Social Work*. CCETSW Paper 3.

_____ (1976) *Values in Social Work*. CCETSW Discussion Paper 13.

Central Statistical Office (1979) *Social Trends. No. 9*. London: HMSO.

Cigno, K. (1979) Where do they all come from? *Community Care* 18.1.79: 26 – 7.

Clare, A. (1976) *Psychiatry in Dissent*. London: Tavistock.

Clarke, J. (1971) An Analysis of Crisis Management by Mental Welfare Officers. *British Journal of Social Work* **1** (1): 27 – 39.

Claydon, C. (1976) Taking Children into Care. *Community Care* (Supplement) October.

Clough, R. (1978) In Residence: Residential Homes in the Community. *Social Work Today* **9** (25): 18.

Creighton, S. J. and Outram, P. J. (1977) *Child Victims of Physical Abuse*. London: NSPCC.

Davies, B. and McLeod, E. (1978) What Use are Integrated Models? *Community Care* 21.6.78: 22 – 3.

Davies, E. M. (1975) *Lets get Moving*. London: Age Concern.

Davis, L. (1978) In Residence – Beyond the Key Worker Concept. *Social Work Today* **9** (19): 17.

DHSS (1974) *Report of an Inquiry into the Care Provided in Relation to Maria Colwell*. London: HMSO.

_____ (1975) *Better Services for the Mentally Ill*. London: HMSO.

_____ (1976a) *A Lifestyle for the Elderly*. DHSS Development Group Report Series.

_____ (1976b) *Foster Care: a Guide to Practice*. London: HMSO.

_____ (1976c) Some Aspects of Residential Care. *Social Work Service* **10** (July): 3 – 17.

_____ (1976d) *Priorities for Health and Personal Social Services in England*. London: HMSO.

_____ (1978) *Review of the Mental Health Act*. London: HMSO.

DHSS/Welsh Office (1977) *Residential Homes for the Elderly: Arrangements for Health Care. A Memorandum of Guidance*. London: HMSO.

Dinnage, R. and Pringle, M. L. K. (1967a) *Foster Care – Facts and Fallacies*. London: Longman/National Children's Bureau.

_____ (1967b) *Residential Care – Facts and Fallacies*. London: Longman/National Children's Bureau.

Draper, J. (1978) How Ennals has Acted on the Act. *Community Care* 6.12.78: 19 – 22.

Dunham, J. (1978) Staff Stress in Residential Work. *Social Work Today* 9 (45): 18 – 20.

Eekelaar, J. (1971) *Family Security and Family Breakdown*. Harmondsworth: Penguin.

Elder, G. (1977) *The Alienated. Growing Old Today*. London: Writers and Readers Publishing Cooperative.

Ennals, D. (1978) The Role of Residential Care. *Social Work Today* 10 (7): 14 – 15.

Evaluation Research Group, University of Sheffield (1977) *The Sheffield Developmental Project on Services for the Mentally Handicapped*. University of Sheffield.

Feldman, L. (1978) *Care Proceedings*. London: Oyez.

Fennell, P. W. H. (1977) The Mental Health Review Tribunal: A Question of Imbalance. *British Journal of Law and Society* 4 (2): 186 – 219.

Foren, R. and Bailey, R. (1968) *Authority in Social Casework*. London: Pergamon.

Fraiberg, S. and Regensburg, J. (1957) *Direct Casework with Children*. Family Service Association of America.

Fraiberg, S. (1959) *The Magic Years*. London: Methuen.

Freeman, M. D. A. (1974) *The Legal Structure*. London: Longman.

Fry, M. (1954) *Old Age Looks at Itself*. London: Churchill Livingstone.

Gibberd, K. (1977) *Home for Life: Residential Care. What Alternatives?* London: Age Concern.

Godek, S. (1977) *Barnado Social Work Papers (2)-Leaving Care*. London: Barnado Publications.

Goffman, E. (1961) *Asylums. Essays on the Social Situation of Mental Patients and Other Inmates*. Harmondsworth: Penguin (1970).

Golan, N. (1969) When is a Client in Crisis? *Social Casework* 50 (7) (July): 389 – 94.

Goldberg, E. M., Mortimer, A., and Williams, B. T. (1970) *Helping the Aged*. London: Allen and Unwin.

Goldberg, E. M. Warburton, R. W., McGuiness, B., and Rowlands, J. H. (1977) Towards Accountability in Social Work: One Year's Intake to an Area Office. *British Journal of Social Work* 7 (3): 257 – 84.

Goldberg, E. M. and Connelly, N. (1978) Reviewing Services for the Old. *Community Care* 6.12.78: 27 – 30.

Goldstein, H. (1973) *Social Work Practice: A Unitary Approach*. University of South Carolina.

Goldstein, J., Freud, A., and Solnit, A. (1973) *Beyond the Best Interests of the Child*. New York: Collier-Macmillan.

Gordon, H. (1978) Observations on Statutory Examinations. *Social Work Today* 9 (42): 24 – 5.

Gostin, L. O. (1975) *A Human Condition. Vol. I*. London: National Association for Mental Health.

Greene, M. R. (1977) *Risk and Insurance* (4th edn.). Cincinatti: South Western Publishing Co.

Greenleigh, A. (1955) Some Psychological Aspects of Aging. *Social Casework* (March): 99 – 106.

Grey, M. (1979) Forcing Old People to Leave their Homes. *Community Care* 8.3.79: 19 – 20.

Gutman, G. M. and Herbert, C. P. (1976) Mortality Rates Among Relocated Extended-Care Patients. *Journal of Gerontology* 31 (3): 352 – 57.

Hadley, R., Webb, A., and Farrell, C. (1975) *Across the Generations*. London: Allen and Unwin.

Hall, J. G. and Mitchell, B. (1978) *Child Abuse – Procedure and Evidence in Juvenile Courts*. Chichester: Barry Rose.

Hall, M. R. P., MacLennan, W. J., and Lye, M. D. W. (1978) *Medical Care of the Elderly*. London: H. M. and M. Publishers.

Hansard Vol. 444, House of Commons (1948). National Assistance Bill, order for second reading: 1603 – 1716.

Harris, D. (1977) Seven Models of Residential Care. *Social Work Today* 9 (1): 19 – 20.

Hazel, N. (1978) Children in Care Should be in Transit. *Community Care* 5.7.78.

Heinicke, C. M. and Westheimer, I. J. (1965) *Brief Separations*. London: Longman.

Heywood, J. and Allen, B. (1971) *Financial Help in Social Work*. Manchester: Manchester University Press.

Hoggett, B. (1976) *Social Work and the Law: Mental Health*. London: Sweet and Maxwell.

_____ (1977) *Social Work and the Law: Parents and Children*. London: Sweet and Maxwell.

Holgate, E. (ed.) (1972) *Communicating with Children*. London: Longman.

Hollis, F. (1964) *Casework: A Psychosocial Therapy*. New York: Random House.

Holman, R. (1966) The Child and the Child Care Officer. *Case Conference* 13 (2): 39 – 43.

Hunt, A. (1978) *The Elderly at Home*. London: HMSO.

Hudson, J. R. (1975) Admission to Care. *Social Work Today* 6 (2): 45 – 8.

Hunter, J. and Ainsworth, F. (1973) *Residential Establishments – the Evolving of Caring Systems*. University of Dundee, Conference Papers.

Ingram, E. (1961) Play and Leisure Time in the Children's Home. *Case Conference* 7 (7): 165 – 69.

Jackson, G. (1971) Authority and the Mental Welfare Officer. *British Journal of Psychiatric Social Work* 9 (1): 22 – 4.

Jehu, D. (1963) *Casework Before Admission to Care*. Association of Child Care Officers: Monograph 1.

Jenkins, R. (1978) The Crisis of Separation. *Social Work Today* 10 (4): 23 – 4.

Jenkins, S. and Norman, E. (1972) *Filial Deprivation and Foster Care*. Columbia: Columbia University Press.

Johnson, M. (1976) That Was Your Life: A Biographical Approach to Later Life. In J. M. A. Munnichs and W. J. A. Van Den Heuvel (eds.) *Dependency or Interdependency in Old Age*. The Hague: Martinus Nijhoff.

Jones, B. (1976) Social Workers at Risk. *Social Work Today* 6 (25): 780 – 82.

Jones, G. M. (1978) *The implementation of policies regarding the use of Local Authority old peoples homes: A study of the perceptions of social service departmental personnel in the Welsh counties*. M.A. dissertation University of Wales (unpublished).

Jones, K. (1972a) The Twenty-Four Steps: An Analysis of Institutional Admission Procedures. *Sociology* 6: 405 – 14.

—— (1972b) *A History of the Mental Health Services*. London: Routledge and Kegan Paul.

—— (1977) The Wrong Target in Mental Health? *New Society* 3.3.77.

Journal of Personality and Social Psychology 20 (3): December 1971: Special Issue on the Risky-Shift.

Kastell, J. (1962) *Casework in Child Care*. London: Routledge and Kegan Paul.

Kay, N. (1970) The Impact of Compulsory Removal of Children on Family Cohesion. *Social Work (G.B.)* (January): 16 – 18.

Kent, E. A. (1963) Role of Admission Stress in Adaptation of Older People in Institutions. *Geriatrics* (February): 133 – 38.

Kushlik, A. and Blunden, R. (1974) *Proposals for the setting up and evaluation of an experimental service for the elderly. A document for discussion.* Wessex Health Care Evaluation and Research Team: Research Report No. 107.

Latane, B. and Darley, J. M. (1970) *The Unresponsive Bystander: Why Doesn't He Help?* Indianopolis: Meredith Corporation.

Lennhoff, F. G. (1967) The Experience of Separation. In *Being Sent Away*. Shotton Hall Publications.

Lewis, B. and Oldfield, C. (1977) *The Maintenance of the Elderly in the Community*. Cicely Northcote Trust.

Lieberman, M. A. (1974) Symposium — Long-Term Care: Research, Policy and Practice. Relocation Research and Social Policy. *The Gerontologist* 14 (6): 494 – 500.

Lindemann, E. (1976) Grief and Grief Management: Some Reflections. *Journal of Pastoral Care* 30 (3).

Litin, E. M. (1956) Mental Reaction to Trauma and Hospitalization in the Aged. *Journal American Medical Association* 162 (17): 515 – 19.

Littner, N. (1956) *Some Traumatic Effects of Separation and Placement*. Child Welfare League of America.

Lowenstein, L. F. (1978) Residential Care for Problem Children — Are We All Going Wrong? *Social Work Today* 9 (23): 11 – 14.

Lowther, C. P. and McLeod, H. M. (1974) Admissions to a Welfare Home. *Health Bulletin* 32 (1): 14 – 18.

Manning, M. (1979) Year of the Child. *Community Care* 15.3.79: 22 – 5.

Marris, P. (1974) *Loss and Change*. London: Routledge and Kegan Paul.

Maslow, A. (1962) *Towards a Psychology of Being*. New Orleans Insight.

Mason, E. M. (1968) The Importance to a Child of his Family. In R. J. N. Tod (ed.) *Children in Care*. London: Longman.

Meacher, M. (1972) *Taken for a Ride*. London: Longman.

MIND (1976) *In-Service Training for Social Work with the Mentally Ill*. London: MIND.

——— (1978) *Press Release on the White Paper*. London: MIND.

Ministry of Health (1966) *Annual Report on the State of Public Health*. London: HMSO.

Monach, J. (1978) A Suitable Case for Compulsory Admission. *Social Work Today* 9 (42): 22 – 4.

Monahan, J. (1978) Prediction Research and the Emergency Commitment of Dangerous Mentally Ill Persons: A Reconsideration. *American Journal of Psychiatry* 135 (2): 198 – 201.

Moore, J. (1976) The Child Client. *Social Work Today* 8 (3): 13 – 15.

Moroney, R. M. (1976) *The Family and the State*. London: Longman.

Moss, S. Z. (1966) How Children Feel about Being Placed Away from

Home. *Children* **13** (4): July/August. Reprinted in Tod, R. J. N. *Disturbed Children*. London: Longman (1968).

National Association of Probation Officers (1977) *Risk − An Analysis of the Problem of Risk in Social Work Practice*. London: NAPO.

NSPCC (1976) *At Risk: An Account of the Work of the Battered Child Research Department*. London: Routledge and Kegan Paul.

Newson, E. (1971) Who am I − where do I come from? *Concern* (NCB) (8): 26 − 7.

Olsen, R. (1977) A New Approach to the Mental Health Emergency. *Social Work Today* **8** (39): 7 − 9.

Oram, E. (1978) Compulsory Admission to Psychiatric Hospital: Legislation and Practice. *Social Work Today* **9** (42): 19 − 21.

Pablo, R. Y. (1977) Intra-institutional Relocation: Its Impact on Long-Term Care Patients. *The Gerontologist* **17** (5): 426 − 35.

Packman, J. (1973) Incidence of Need. In J. Stroud (ed.) *Services for Children and their Families*. Oxford: Pergamon.

Parad, H. (1965) *Crisis Intervention*. London: FSAA.

Parker, R. A. (1978) Foster Care in Context. *Adoption and Fostering* **93** (3).

Parkes, C. M. (1975) *Bereavement: Studies of Grief in Adult Life*. Harmondsworth: Penguin.

Pattie, A. H. and Gilleard, C. J. (1978) Admission and Adjustment of Residents in Homes for the Elderly. *Journal of Epidemiology and Community Health* **32**: 212 − 14.

Payne, C. (1977) In Residence. Caring for the Care Givers. *Social Work Today* **8** (15): 14 − 15.

Payne, L. (1976) How Matthew Lost his Mum. *Community Care* 4.2.76.

Pearson, G. (1977) *The Deviant Imagination*. London: Macmillan.

Personal Social Services Council (1975) *Living and Working in Residential Homes*. London: PSSC.

—— (1977) *Residential Care Reviewed*. London: PSSC.

—— (1979) *Comments on 'A Happier Old Age'*. London: PSSC.

Personal Social Services Research Unit, University of Kent (1979) *Kent Community Care Project*. Paper No. 30: University of Kent.

Picardie, M. (1970) The Identity of Social Work. *Social Work Today* **1** (7): 37 − 42.

Pincus, A. and Minahan, A. (1973) *Social Work Practice: Model and Method*. London: F. E. Peacock.

Pitt, B. (1974) *Psychogeriatrics: An Introduction to the Psychiatry of Old Age*. London: Churchill Livingstone.

Plank, D. (1977) *Caring for the Elderly. Report of a study of various means of caring for dependent elderly people in 8 London Boroughs*. Greater London Council.

_____ (1979) quoted in *Social Work Today* 10 (37).

Pope, P. (1978) Admissions to Residential Homes for the Elderly. *Social Work Today* 9 (44): 12 – 16.

Post, F. (1965) *The Clinical Psychiatry of Later Life*. London: Pergamon.

_____ (1974) Foreword to J. A. Whitehead: *Psychiatric Disorders in Old Age*. Aylesbury: H. M. and M. Publishers.

Pringle, M. L. K. (1971) *Deprivation and Education*. London: Longman/National Children's Bureau.

_____ (1975) *The Needs of Children*. London: Hutchinson.

Pugh, E. (1968) *Social Work in Child Care*. London: Routledge and Kegan Paul.

Rapoport, L. (1965) The State of Crisis: Some Theoretical Considerations. In H. J. Parad (ed.) *Crisis Intervention*. New York: FSAA.

Rees, S. J. (1976) Defining Moral Worthiness: Grounds for Intervention in Social Work. *Social Work Today* 7 (7): 203 – 06.

Rees, S. (1978) *Social Work Face to Face*. London: Edward Arnold.

Reith, D. (1975) I wonder if you can help me . . .? *Social Work Today* 6 (3): 66 – 9.

RCA jointly with BASW (1976) How Can Residential and Field Social Workers Co-operate? *Social Work Today* 7 (12): 346 – 48.

Rich, J. (1968) *Interviewing Children and Adolescents*. London: Macmillan.

Roberts, A. (1976) Response to Innovation – Government Policy Towards the Mentally Disordered. In R. Olsen (ed.) *Differential Approaches to Social Work with the Mentally Disordered*. Birmingham: BASW.

Roberts, R. W. and Nee, R. H. (1970) *Theories of Social Casework*. Chicago: University of Chicago Press.

Robertson, J. and J. (1968) *Children in Brief Separation – John, Kate, etc.* Concorde Film Council.

Rokeach, M. (1973) *The Nature of Human Values*. New York: The Free Press.

Rosin, A. J. (1966) Complications of Illness in Geriatric Patients in Hospital. *Journal of Chronic Disease* 19: 307 – 13.

Rowe, J. and Lambert, L. (1973) *Children Who Wait: A Study of Children Needing Substitute Families*. ABAA.

Rutter, M. (1972) *Maternal Deprivation Reassessed*. Harmondsworth: Penguin.

Saul, S. (1974) *Aging: An Album of People Growing Old*. Chichester: John Wiley.

Sayer, P., Forbes, D., Newman, P., and Jameson, T. (1976) Positive Planning for Children in Care. *Social Work Today* 8 (2): 9 – 11.

Shanas, E., Townsend, P., Wedderburn, D., Friis, H., Milkay, A., and Stehower, J. (1968) *Old People in Three Industrial Societies.* London: Routledge and Kegan Paul.

Shaw, I. and Walton, R. (1978) Transition to Residence, School of Social Work, University of Cardiff 1977. Quoted in P. Pope: Admissions to Residential Homes for the Elderly. *Social Work Today* **9** (44): 12 – 16.

Shaw, M. and Lebens, K. (1978) *Substitute Family Care: Vol. II What Shall We Do With the Children?* London: ABAFA.

Siegler, M. and Osmond, H. (1974) *Models of Madness, Models of Medicine.* London: Macmillan.

Smaldino, A. (1975) The Importance of Hope in the Casework Relationship. *Social Casework* **56** (6): 328 – 33.

Smith, J. (1975) How To Get Service or at Least Get By. *Social Work Today* **6** (3): 70 – 2.

Specht, H. and Vickery, A. (eds.) (1977) *Integrating Social Work Methods.* London: Allen and Unwin.

Stanton, B. R. and Exton Smith, A. N. (1970) *A Longitudinal Study of the Dietary Needs of Elderly Women.* London: King Edward's Hospital Fund.

Stevenson, O. (1963a) Reception into Care – its Meaning for all Concerned. *Case Conference* **10** (4): 110 – 14.

—— (1963b) The Understanding Caseworker. *New Society* 1.8.63.

—— (1978a) *Reception into Care – Case Example.* In CCETSW Study No. 1. *Good Enough Parenting.*

—— (1978b) *Ageing. A Professional Perspective.* London: Age Concern.

Strongman, K. T. (1979) *Psychology for the Paramedical Professions.* London: Croom Helm.

Thomas, J. (1977) Comment – Communicating with Children. *Social Work Today* **8** (25): 1.

Timms, N. and Itzin, F. (1961) The Role of the Child Care Officer. *British Journal of Psychiatric Social Work* **6** (2): 74 – 83.

Timms, N. (1962) *Casework in the Child Care Service.* London: Butterworth.

Tobin, S. S. and Lieberman, M. A. (1976) *Last Home for the Aged.* California: Jossey-Bass.

Tod, R. J. N. (ed.) (1968) *Disturbed Children.* London: Longman.

Townsend, P. (1970) *The Fifth Social Service.* London: Fabian Society.

Trasler, G. (1960) In Place of Parents. London: Routledge and Kegan Paul.

—— (1968) The Consequences of Separation. *Mental Health* **21** (3): 1962, Reprinted in R. J. N. Tod (ed.) *Children in Care.* London: Longman.

Trieschman, A. E., Whittaker, J. K., and Brendtro, L. K. (1969) *The Other 23 Hours*. Chicago: Aldine.

Triseliotis, J. (1979) When the Bonds are Thicker than Blood. *Community Care* 28.6.79: 17 – 20.

Turner, F. J. (ed.) (1968) *Differential Diagnosis and Treatment in Social Work*. New York: The Free Press.

Utting, B. (1977) Residential Care – The End or the Beginning. *Social Work Today* 9 (7): 14 – 17.

Vann, J. (1971) The Child as Client of the Social Services Department. *British Journal of Social Work* 1 (2): 209 – 24.

Webb, A. (1975) Working Paper A. In *Living and Working in Residential Homes*. London: Personal Social Services Council.

Weed, L. L. (1969) *Medical Records, Medical Education and Patient Care*. Case Western Reserve University Press.

Whittaker, J. A. (1974) *Social Treatment: An Approach to Interpersonal Helping*. Chicago: Aldine.

Wicks, M. (1978) *Old and Cold. Hypothermia and Social Policy*. London: Heinemann.

Williams, A. C. (jr.) and Heins, R. M. (1971) *Risk Management and Insurance* (2nd edn.). New York: McGraw-Hill.

Winnicott, C. (1964) *Child Care and Social Work*. Bristol: Bookstall Publications.

—— (1977) Face to Face with Children. *Social Work Today* 8 (26): 7 – 11.

Winnicott, D. W. (1971) *Playing and Reality*. Harmondsworth: Penguin.

Yawney, B. A. and Slover, D. L. (1973) Relocation of the Elderly. *Social Work* 18 (3): 86 – 95.

Younghusband, E. (ed.) (1965) *Social Work with Families*. London: Allen and Unwin.

Young People's Working Group (1977) *Who Cares? Young People in Care Speak Out*. London: National Children's Bureau.

Name Index

Figure in italics refers to bibliographical references

Subject Index

221